SIGNS OF DISABILITY

CRIP: NEW DIRECTIONS IN DISABILITY STUDIES

General Editors: Michael Bérubé, Robert McRuer, and Ellen Samuels

Committed to generating new paradigms and attending to innovative interdisciplinary shifts, the Crip: New Directions in Disability Studies series focuses on cutting-edge developments in the field, with interest in exploratory analyses of disability and globalization, ecotheory, new materialisms, affect theory, performance studies, postcolonial studies, and trans theory.

Signs of Disability

Stephanie L. Kerschbaum

NEW YORK UNIVERSITY PRESS

New York

NEW YORK UNIVERSITY PRESS
New York
www.nyupress.org

References to Internet websites (URLs) were accurate at the time of writing. Neither the author nor New York University Press is responsible for URLs that may have expired or changed since the manuscript was prepared.

Library of Congress Cataloging-in-Publication Data
Names: Kerschbaum, Stephanie L., 1977– author.
Title: Signs of disability / Stephanie L. Kerschbaum.
Description: New York : New York University Press, [2022] |
Series: Crip: new directions in disability studies |
Includes bibliographical references and index.
Identifiers: LCCN 2022002125 | ISBN 9781479811144 (hardback ; alk. paper) |
ISBN 9781479811168 (paperback ; alk. paper) | ISBN 9781479811175 (ebook other) |
ISBN 9781479811182 (ebook)
Subjects: LCSH: People with disabilities. | Sociology of disability.
Classification: LCC HV1568 .K48 2022 | DDC 362.4—dc23/eng/20220224
LC record available at https://lccn.loc.gov/2022002125

New York University Press books are printed on acid-free paper, and their binding materials are chosen for strength and durability. We strive to use environmentally responsible suppliers and materials to the greatest extent possible in publishing our books.

Manufactured in the United States of America

10 9 8 7 6 5 4 3 2 1

Also available as an ebook

To Jamie, Rosemary, and Rhys,
and to my mother,
for everything

CONTENTS

Introduction

Signs of Disability

As I have lived a life as a deaf person, I have moved from ignoring disability as much as possible to framing disability as something that only mattered in special circumstances to recognizing disability as mattering everywhere and everywhen. Signs of disability are all around us, even if we don't always know how to pay attention to them. Take deafness as an example. Even though deafness is sometimes referred to as an invisible disability, ubiquitous signs disclose deafness: behind-the-ear hearing aids emitting high-pitched feedback; hands moving in air producing sign language; the close physical proximity and connection required by pro-tactile ASL; the multisensory environments created by "Deaf Space" architectural design; the habit of making sure someone has turned their gaze in your direction before speaking; yellow diamond-shaped "Deaf Person in Area" road signs. All of these signs have appeared to me in different ways and at different times. I write now as a white, middle-aged, deaf woman and academic who has been immersed in disability studies for almost fifteen years and who has built relationships with a range of deaf and disabled people, experiences that have taught me how to notice deafness. While I was born deaf, I was not born noticing deafness. My attention to deafness has been shaped over time as I have moved through the world as part of an ongoing and dynamic process that Karen Barad describes as coming to know the world even as "we are *of* the world."[1] Deafness is not a material thing I can point to, but it emerges materially through how I perceive particular objects and cues and behaviors, as well as how others respond to and engage with me.

My attention to disability and deafness shifts, sometimes dramatically, in different contexts and settings and at different times and places. When I attended new-student orientation before the start of my first year of college at Ohio State, I tried to convince the office for disability services that I did not need sign language interpreting or captioning for my classes. After pressure from OSU's interpreting coordinator and from my parents, I agreed to "just try it." And even when I grudgingly acknowledged how much of a difference interpreting and captioning made for me, I still felt that my disability did not matter that much and if it did matter, it was only under very specific circumstances. It was not until after I had finished graduate school and started an academic career that I really confronted the mattering of disability in my life and work. I was in my late twenties and writing my first book under the pressure of the tenure clock. Feeling intense anxiety about my professional future, I knew I needed to publish. In what I might characterize as desperation, I finally caved and followed advice I had received from multiple colleagues: I wrote about my deafness in an article. I had resisted these suggestions for a long time because I wanted to believe my disability had nothing to do with the research I was doing. However, once I did this work, nearly every reader commented on how powerful my discussion of disability was and how helpful they found it to my theorizing.[2] While I was heartened by this praise, it nevertheless made me feel uneasy. I was accustomed to not wanting my disability to be the center of attention, of not wanting it to matter, and this praise made me worry about what it meant that it seemed to matter so much to everyone else.

Now, of course I knew my disability mattered. My undergraduate experiences with accommodations led me to immediately request captioning and interpreting when I started graduate school. When I went on the academic job market for the first time, I made interpreting requests for every interview because I did not want to risk being in the awkward and possibly job-offer-threatening situation of having someone I could not understand ask me a question.[3] Various tensions I felt around whether and how to disclose my deafness were inflected by the normativity of my other readily apparent identifications as a white, cisgender woman in a heterosexual partnership. When I received a job offer, I made clear that I would need regular access to sign language interpreting, and over time, I integrated accommodations into more and more arenas of my academic life. And yet, throughout all this change, I did not *want* my deafness to matter. I was deeply invested in maintaining my sense that at least in my writing, in my scholarship, in many areas of my life, it did not matter that much.

I was wrong.

And I came to this realization only gradually, over time, and as the direct outcome of the material circumstances of my professional life. My tenure-track years were dominated by conference experiences with uneven interpreting services that largely provided just a veneer of accessibility. One way I responded to conferences' inaccessibility involved significant behind-the-scenes labor in which I created detailed schedules for each session at a conference, searched for the email addresses for all the panelists, and sent carefully crafted, rhetorically invitational, gratitude-laden, and (I hoped) persuasive requests for them to bring extra copies of their scripts that I could read from during their presentation.[4] The time, energy, and organization this work required of me meant I could not do it for every conference. And even when I did, I could never fully predict whether those I contacted would be willing to provide a script, remember to bring one, or even respond to my email. This led me to disability studies sessions because their panelists frequently built accessibility into their talks. I learned to make predictions about which panels would be most likely to have speakers share access copies and planned my attendance accordingly.

Having access copies meant that I would still be able to participate in some capacity at a conference even if I did not laboriously contact everyone ahead of time, and even if the interpreting was subpar.[5] Problems with the provision of sign language interpreting were common situations for me and for many other deaf academics, not only because relatively few people, groups, or organizations factored access and accommodation costs into their event budgets but because, as Teresa Blankmeyer Burke explains in "Choosing Accommodations," there is a wide continuum of sign language, from ASL to Signed English, and interpreters have "variable levels of skill and proficiency" that most event organizers are not poised to effectively assess or evaluate.[6] The frequent resistance I experienced around the cost of accommodations[7] led me to collaborate with others to create additional forms of access as well as to seek out low-cost or cost-neutral options. In this way, because of the mattering of how I process sound and visual input, I was repeatedly connected to disability studies scholarship and other disabled scholars even though I did not—for a long time—understand their work as directly relevant to my own academic and professional interests.

These ongoing efforts around conference accessibility involved many forms of collaboration and coalition and, along with my experiences of smoother paths of access to disability studies, were part of a process of building an attentional and perceptual apparatus for disability: a way of looking for and perceiving disability as well as for theorizing my own lived experiences. The account I have shared here shows disability taking on different valences and significances over the course of moving in and through particular environments with different people at different times. It is also an account in which I am working to make disability available to you—readers of this book—in textual form, drawing on various means and resources for doing so. These efforts undergird the questions motivating this book: How does disability, through embodied, material interactions of all kinds, become available for perception and meaning? How does disability emerge as something to which we can attend? How does disability matter?

One site for exploring the mattering of disability is interpersonal interaction, encounters during which people engage in a process that I have elsewhere theorized as "marking difference."[8] In marking difference, people display and interpret markers of difference in both conscious and nonconscious ways as they position themselves against and alongside others. Markers of difference are emergent, dynamic, and relational rhetorical cues that include forms of embodied and enminded presence, material accoutrements, linguistic and paralinguistic utterances, behaviors, practices, and more. In the stories I have shared about myself thus far, numerous cues have conveyed information to you about who I am and how this text might be interpreted or understood. This book's materialization, whether you are perusing a screen or a manuscript page, listening to a screen reader, holding a bound book, feeling a Braille interface, listening to the book be read aloud by another, or engaging with the text through a wide range of other means, is also part of how readers come to understand me and this text vis-à-vis deafness, disability, and difference.

While it can be tempting to imagine disability as a narrower classification of difference, and then again to think of deafness as a narrower classification of disability, these categories actually do not work this way. Deafness is as infinite as disability is as infinite as difference. All are dynamic, emergent, and relational capacities for moving and being that interact and materially and discursively constitute reality and everyday lived experience. Rather than situating these categories as sets and subsets of one another, it is more useful to think of them as ever-expanding capacities for sociomaterial emergence. Any attempt to define deafness, which most often happens textually through reference to a big-D, little-d distinction that distinguishes between deafness as a cultural identification and the impairment of being unable to hear sounds, ultimately fails.[9] While this distinction in some contexts does important and useful work, it is inadequate for describing many deaf people's experiences, and it can presume a totality and coherence that have not been reflected in any grouping of deaf people I have encountered. Once we start trying to define deafness or disability or difference, they slip out of our grasp and elude definition or determination. They commingle and associate and entangle with the intricacies of lived experience, of changing worlds and bodies and technologies and relations, ultimately becoming what Ellen Samuels has termed "fantasies of identification" that exceed and conflict with existing ontologies.[10]

Notions of deafness and disability—my own and those reflected back to me by others—were consequential for just about every choice I made early in my career, not just those involving access and accommodation. In my work studying markers of difference and as I have developed the concept of signs of disability, I have noticed that both involve investments in certain kinds of selves. For instance, as I listened to students interacting in a writing classroom, I came to understand that their willingness to participate in an interaction was constituted through their display and uptake of markers of difference.[11] When students recognized the self that others showed back to them interactionally, they were willing to respond and engage. Similar investments are apparent in my early-career resistance to writing about myself in my scholarship. Somehow, it felt different—scarier, more threatening—to make such disclosures in writing than to navigate them in everyday interpersonal space. This is perhaps related to the fact that I have developed strategies for making people comfortable as they interact with me in person, including using humor and smiling a lot, which are behaviors also inflected by my whiteness and gender. In an interpersonal encounter, I experience possibilities for change and relationship building in ways that written texts can foreclose. In addition, given the number of encounters I have had with people who have discredited my authority, when I did not know who might read a written text, those disclosures felt threatening. This threat took on salience for me because of how much my work involves listening to aural conversations using my residual hearing, extremely strong hearing aid amplification, written transcripts, and collaboration. During my pretenure period, I worried intensely about how my deafness might matter to those in positions to evaluate or respond to my work.

While fears around disqualification have subsided somewhat with the publication and critical reception of my first book, they have not left me entirely, and indeed, they continue to shift and morph in ways that I am always coming to know. For instance, early in the process of working on this book, I conducted a research interview with a blind faculty member who requested the phone as an interview modality. Because I cannot understand spoken conversation without a visual complement, I registered with an online relay service that would caption the call and used a video camera to record myself conducting the interview. However, only after questioning from others did I wrestle with a significant omission in the analytic scene: I did not record in real time how I actually accessed this conversation. I had been entirely focused on the audio coming through the phone as the most important way to access the interviewee's words. Consequently, I barely considered that the words scrolling on my laptop through the relay interface were just as essential as the phone's audio to the unfolding interaction.[12]

If I am really honest with myself—and it has taken me years to even acknowledge this to myself, much less share it publicly in this book—the truth is that even if I had thought prior to the interview about recording the internet relay captioning in real time, I would have had strong resistance to it, might not have been willing to do it, or might only have done it extremely reluctantly and with great trepidation. Internet relay captions are rarely as accurate as I desire, and transcript infelicities are common. Having the differences between the aural and visual modes of this interview be front and center in the research process would have made apparent some of the gaps in my access to the scene, gaps that have only very recently come to be theorized as potentially productive and generative sites of meaning making rather than as deficits or problems.[13]

My own focus on deafness and disability (and to a lesser extent gender) as a threat to my professional identity also underscores the role that whiteness has played in my life: my energy for access labor in my career has been supported and sustained by the ease with which I navigate predominantly white professional settings. That race can be backgrounded in my conscious awareness has meant that it has not always been an aspect of my identity around which I have been vigilant. Over my life and career, I have had to work to make race—and my whiteness in particular—central to my everyday noticing. The mattering of deafness and disability, then, is always taking shape and changing as I come into (different) awareness of my embodied materiality through various personal and professional encounters. This mattering changes as I experience the boundaries and borders of deafness and disability as an ever-shifting terrain that I can never fully understand or map out. In thinking about how deafness and disability matter, I refer both to their material substance and presence and to how that mattering and presence take on meaning, weight, and significance.

To materialize signs of disability is a never-ending inquiry into who and what is (un)recognized and in what configurations. No two experiences of deafness are the same, and even my own deafness is different across time and space. I have found myself wanting to tear and rip and crush into pulp the distinctions, lines, barriers, boundaries that delineate deafness and disability and then I want to make that pulp into paper again and then I want to tear it up again and remake it again and on and on. Those acts of tearing, cutting, crushing, and then remaking and reshaping? They are the everyday mattering of disability. This everyday mattering suggests an approach to disability as a continual, protracted, effort-laden, and "frictioned"[14] process of seeking both recognition[15] and moments of unrecognizability.[16] These explorations ask how complex relations—entanglements—among beings, environments, materials, and meaning enable the emergence and perceptibility of disability. They ask what it means for disability to appear, to be perceptible or imperceptible, to emerge as what Julie Avril Minich has suggested as a critical methodology[17] or what Tobin Siebers has called a body of knowledge,[18] and they ask how boundaries around social encounters and environments point to disability. These are all questions about the mattering of disability.

My response is to theorize signs of disability as perceptual cues that point to the presence or emergence of disability, a definition that recalls and extends my earlier work on marking difference. In my book *Toward a New Rhetoric of Difference*, I defined markers of difference as "contextually embedded rhetorical cues that signal the presence of difference between one or more interlocutors."[19] This definition emphasizes marking as happening in situated performances involving real-time synchronous interaction, approaching difference as interactionally emergent, changing over the course of an interaction, and in relation with others. However, for reasons I will explain in more detail below, markers of difference largely focus attention on discursive forms of marking that can make it difficult to account for material objects and artifacts that also participate in these interactional scenes. Extending markers of difference, then, signs of disability emphasize the entanglement of sensory input, everyday reality, and interpretive relations that lead to the emergence of phenomena. This framework does not constrain the signaling of disability to readily recognized communicative forms, and it takes seriously the agency of all matter.

I have learned to understand material agency through multiple academic threads stitching together stories of human and material interconnections that have helped me think through relations among perceivers and what is perceived. A key thread comes from Indigenous theorist Robin Wall Kimmerer, whose work centers story while refusing typical disciplinary divides in scientific inquiry that separate lived experience and knowledge building. In "Asters and Goldenrod," Kimmerer describes fields and meadows "embroidered with drifts of golden yellow and pools of deeper purple, a masterpiece." Painting a portrait of these flowers in words, Kimmerer says, "Alone, each is a botanical superlative. Together, the visual effect is stunning: Purple and gold, the heraldic colors of the king and queen of the meadow, a regal procession in complementary colors. I just wanted to know why." But a botany adviser tells her that question is not science: "He told me that science was not about beauty, not about the embrace between plants and humans."[20] When Kimmerer headed to college and studied plant biology, the scientific approach her professors taught her insisted on "separating the observer from the observed, and the observed from the observer," which relegated questions about why two plants were beautiful together to a realm of subjectivity. However, Kimmerer shows that there are explanations for this beauty that can only be understood through the connections between the scientific knowledge from her professional training and the traditional knowledges she grew up with: "Why are they beautiful together? It is a phenomenon simultaneously material and spiritual, for which we need all wavelengths, for which we need depth perception. When I stare too long at the world with science eyes, I see an afterimage of traditional knowledge. Might science and traditional knowledge be purple and yellow to one another? Might they be goldenrod and asters? We see the world more fully when we use both."[21]

The complementarity between science and traditional knowledges that Kimmerer urges us to recognize can be woven with Karen Barad's account of agential realism in *Meeting the Universe Halfway*. Barad's theory, as does Kimmerer's story, stresses the imbrication of observer and observed. Unlike Kimmerer, Barad does so with a vocabulary taken not from plant biology and Indigenous teaching but from quantum physics.

Barad's account of agential realism imbricates ethics, ontology, and epistemology to stress a responsibility to take seriously the world's materiality as beings of all kinds move in and around and through it. "Intra-action" is a neologism Barad uses to describe "the mutual constitution of entangled agencies."[22] This mutual constitution means that they do not exist as distinct entities that come together (entangle) but rather emerge through intra-action. Matter is not "a fixed substance" but "a stabilizing and destabilizing process of iterative intra-activity" in which phenomena emerge through intra-actions between apparatuses of observation and the world's materiality.[23] These phenomena do not themselves constitute reality: they are the outcome of the intra-actions between observer and observed. Observational apparatuses enact what Barad calls "agential cuts" that make determinate some properties of the phenomenon while leaving others indeterminate.

Stories (or narratives—I use these terms somewhat interchangeably in this book) can then be understood as outcomes of agential cuts enacted by perceptual apparatuses intra-acting with reality. As such, they offer instances where "matter and meaning meet in a very literal sense"[24] as the world is given an account. In Barad's theory, intra-acting agencies point to the "agential" in agential realism, while "realism" refers to the responsibility of "providing accurate descriptions of that reality of which we are a part and with which we intra-act."[25] As a performative account, agential realism takes "thinking, observing, and theorizing as practices of engagement with and as part of, the world in which we have our being."[26] Not all of our practices of engagement, however, as both Barad and Kimmerer would argue, are equally valuable or useful. As Barad puts it, "Explanations of various phenomena and events that do not take account of material, as well as discursive, constraints will fail to provide empirically adequate accounts (not any story will do)."[27]

Storying is an important means of building theory and engaging with the world, as Kimmerer teaches. Alongside Kimmerer, I have learned from a wide range of story-theorists, many in my field of writing studies, including Christina Cedillo, V. Jo Hsu, Lisa King, Rose Gubele, and Joyce Rain Anderson, Aja Martinez, Katherine McKittrick, Malea Powell, Andrea Riley-Mukavetz, Tanya Titchkosky, Victor Villanueva, and Remi Yergeau.[28] These theorists draw on a range of minoritized story-traditions to resist dominant accounts that elide much of the world's materiality. In a critique of the way posthumanist and "new" materialist thinking often universalizes ontology, Chad Shomura suggests instead Jane Bennett's concept of an "onto-*story*" as one means by which materialist scholarship might engage "the difficult labor of navigating multiple ontologies, amplifying minor connections across racial, gender, species, and material lines in order to challenge the powers that be while offering positive visions of other worlds."[29] What I hear as I tangle my fingers through all of these threads is the importance of listening to the world, ensuring that our stories are accountable to the world around us and to the world always coming-into-existence as we move in relation with others. To tell a story is a means of enacting an observation, of making an agential cut that draws boundaries around a phenomenon. Narratives, in other words, materialize disability.

Materializing disability is a boundary-making process that is never complete. Disability is always shifting, contingent on circumstances, contexts, and particular experiences, relationships, and bodily arrangements. Its meanings are not attached to particular words or configurations—even as I repeatedly use the word "disability" throughout this book, it operates as what Barad calls "an ongoing performance of the world in its differential dance of intelligibility and unintelligibility."[30] In this dance, this concert, this riotous cacophony, "part of the world becomes determinately bounded and propertied in its emergent intelligibility to another part of the world, while lively matterings, possibilities, and impossibilities are reconfigured."[31] My thinking about signs of disability is likewise capacious, interested in the ways that they materialize in complex and dynamic processes of mattering and coming-to-matter.

This dynamism and complex mattering might be illustrated with the sign for disability in American Sign Language (the only sign language I am conversant in). To communicate disability in ASL involves fingerspelling the letters "D" and "A" with the dominant signing hand.[32] This sign for disability takes influence from relatively arbitrary features of the English word (its first letter, for instance) but is otherwise an abstract signifier that does little to engage with disability as a concept. In contrast, ASL signs that name specific disabilities are more physically referential. The sign for deaf in ASL is an outstretched index finger moving either from mouth to ear or from ear to mouth;[33] the sign for blind involves a claw-shaped V handshape moving toward the eyes;[34] the sign for a wheelchair user is to use both hands to imitate the movement of self-propelling a wheelchair.[35] Even signs for less directly embodied concepts such as neurodivergence point to and reference signers' bodyminds[36] in much more direct ways than does this sign for disability. An early reviewer of this manuscript wondered whether this move to abstraction might be a euphemistic one. While I can only speculate on this point, I understand the abstraction embedded in fingerspelling D-A as a response to the challenge of encompassing a wide range of different experiences and bodyminds, and that a similar abstraction might even be more desirable in some cases to offset the tight links sometimes suggested by more embodied-referential signs that might seem to link some disability experiences—such as "neurodivergence" and "autism"—with particular locations on the body. I am here grateful to Margaret Price's thinking on the imbrication of body and mind for challenging easy links between mental disability and the brain,[37] which could usefully inform the development of new ASL signs that might do different conceptual work. However, while I want to recognize the dynamic potential sometimes available in abstraction, the decision to abstract the ASL sign for disability by pointing to English letters does little to convey anything about what disability might mean, be, or do in the world beyond its relationship to the English word. Its meaning is shaped through agential cuts enacted by perceivers—by the stories that emerge around it and with it and through it.

Perceptibility is central to my account of signs of disability, as I have thought about how disability makes itself and is made perceptible with all kinds of cues. While "in/visible disability" and, to a lesser extent, "nonvisible disability" remain perhaps the most common terms for indicating differences between those disabilities that are assumed to be readily interpreted on the basis of material presences and those that are not so readily available for perception, these terms have been critiqued for overemphasizing visual perception and thus eliding many ways that disability might materialize through other kinds of sensory input. I hope the broader term "perceptibility" will also support attention to the ways that different forms of embodied and enminded presence, including race and ethnicity, gender, and sexuality, matter to disability's emergence. Through "perceptibility" I acknowledge the work that observational apparatuses—what I will call in this book perceptual apparatuses—do in intra-acting with the world to produce material phenomena. In so doing, "perceptibility" can resist the idea that there is a world out there waiting to be found when that world is actually always in the process of intra-actively becoming.

Throughout this book I turn often to story to enact my responsibility to tell better accounts of the world. As material-discursive practices that enact agential cuts and delineate boundaries between self and other, between interior and exterior, narrative is a methodological practice for realizing the imbrication of epistemology, ontology, and ethics—of our relationships with all of the world's materiality. Put another way, story is a way to take materiality seriously. Stories work on and through us. They move us. They are everyday and mundane—as are practices of being raced, gendered, sexed, and disabled, which also/often happen through story. They are central to processes of being (mis)recognized and dis-identified as well as to what Remi Yergeau has called "resonance," "an interbodily knowing, a betweenity that pervades."[38] Repeated, recurrent encounters with stories that enact agential cuts between "self" and "other" and create and break down different boundaries have consequences; they *matter*. These intra-actions effect change in us and in our world. One particularly obdurate iterative story circulates around cure, which has been taken up in several recent disability studies texts: Eli Clare's *Brilliant Imperfection*, Alison Kafer's *Feminist, Queer, Crip*, Eunjung Kim's *Curative Violence*, and Jaipreet Virdi's *Hearing Happiness*.[39]

Each of these books traces the effects and outcomes of repeated, persistent, insistent encounters with stories fixated on cure, on erasing disability, on imagining futures without disability. The curative story, which of course is not just *one* story but *many stories*, layered and entangled and thickening and solidifying and loosening and chipping and repeating, is a continually morphing phenomenon with different resonances and acoustics at different times and places and with different audiences. It is through these intra-actions—with reality and with story—that we access the disclosures made by, in, and through the world.

Essential to the work of story and to the framework of signs of disability is the point that stories are material, and their materiality is significant to their emergence, circulation, and consequence. Therí Pickens's literary-phenomenological discussion of Suheir Hammad's poetry emphasizes this materiality, acknowledging Hammad's embodiment, the fragility of breathing, its entanglement with her lived experience as Palestinian and Black and female and finally, how that embodied knowledge emerges in Hammad's poetic structure and arrangement. Pickens's analysis touches on the lyric arrangement, the breathing patterns required to say the poem's words, and the representation of text on the page.[40] The materiality of story becomes especially apparent when we attend to composing practices that cannot be separated from the body, such as hands spinning and twisting and bending in space and time, as Rebecca Sanchez argues. In working through what she calls "interdimensional translation," or "the new modes of being together that emerge when semantic content cannot be separated from a human body signifying," Sanchez highlights the materiality of language and of the everyday disclosures enacted by and through material texts and objects.[41]

Not only are narratives produced by moving and mattering material bodies, but they are also material artifacts, whether recorded onto cassette tapes, saved as digital files on a hard drive, handwritten in journals, typed on sheets of paper, flickering pixels on an e-reader, tucked into a filing cabinet, buried in the recesses of an archive, or bound into a physical book. This production of narrative and its movement in and out of different material forms always occurs within various social configurations and at particular temporal junctures. Consequently, narratives are highly situated and contextualized, as a long history of scholarship in sociolinguistics and linguistic anthropology has documented.[42] The distinct traditions of storying and approaches to narrative that I have drawn upon at different points in my career and in this introduction all entangle in the definitions of "narrative" and "story" that inform this book. I will toggle between these two terms somewhat intentionally because I have been influenced by a wide range of interdisciplinary approaches for making the world's materiality and lived experiences available to others. For me, narratives and stories are emergent intra-actions shaped by myriad factors, including the conditions of their production, authorial presence and bodyminds made available for noticing in various ways, social interactions, and material-discursive surrounds. These intra-actions lead to narrative possibilities at particular moments, and they consequentially influence how narratives appear and circulate as well as what agential cuts the narratives enact as they intra-act with various perceptual apparatuses.

I use this understanding of narrative and story to deepen an understanding of signs of disability and their agential practices. Four core concepts each animate a chapter of this book. In chapter 1, I consider how perceptual apparatuses are built, taking up dominant and disabled practices of attention—what I theorize through *dis*-attention, an intentionally awkward neologism—that materialize disability through intra-actions as perceptual apparatuses entangle with the world's materiality. *Dis*-attentions of all kinds shape everyday experiences of navigating spaces, times, and encounters, but individual and collective perceptions are not the only factors that influence how and what we notice. Signs of disability are always disclosing, that is, playing an active role in the making of meaning. The world's materiality, including of bodyminds and of the processes by which bodyminds observe and describe the world, is an active, intra-acting participant in disability's materialization.

In chapter 2, I consider how the world discloses to us and what this might mean as we learn to attend to the world's materiality. This chapter shows the need for better stories of disability through the accumulation of stories about a yellow, diamond-shaped "Deaf Person in Area" sign that appeared in my neighborhood, and that has stuck with and changed me as I have written this book. Over the course of many encounters with this sign, it disclosed in different ways. The collective stories shared about this sign emphasize that its disclosures are themselves shaped by both dominant and disabled *dis*-attentions enacted by observers and their perceptual practices learned over lifetimes of moving in the world. This imbrication between ethics, ontology, and epistemology—what Barad terms an "ethico-onto-epistem-ology"—extends figurations of disability that do not go far enough in considering disability's various ontologies.

To consider an ethico-onto-epistemology is to stress the links between materiality and meaning. In like fashion, attention to storying across a wide range of encounters reinforces their specificity and materiality: stories are always told at specific times within particular arrangements, and their materiality is an active participant in processes of meaning making and interpretation. The stories I have found myself saying aloud, writing down, returning to, and revising as I have moved this book into existence have led me to understand the importance of what, in chapter 3, I discuss as a process of disabling. "Disabling" in its everyday use can refer both to the process of breaking something so that it no longer functions and to the experience of becoming disabled or identifying as disabled. This latter definition has been used by scholars across an interdisciplinary range to highlight growing recognition of disability in a variety of ways.[43] I build on this work to suggest disabling as a means whereby disabled forms of *dis*-attention intra-act and work toward better accounts of disability.

In addition to telling better stories of disability through processes of disabling, it is also important to understand dispersal, or how stories come to circulate, which is the focus of chapter 4. In most mainstream contexts, disability is (still) most readily available for perception through dominant *dis*-attentions that take up and circulate some accounts and some signs of disability more than others. Dispersing shows that an account of signs of disability and their functions must also integrate an understanding of how they move. Joining the other core concepts of this book—disabled and dominant *dis*-attentions, the world's material disclosures, and processes of disabling—dispersing supports a robust account of how narratives emerge and take shape.

* * *

This book is an intervention in practices of knowledge production. The process of identifying a research question and developing a project is not separable from the end result that comes to circulate and that you are now reading. When I was writing my first book and developing the concept of marking difference, I was analyzing data generated in a classroom study. During that project, I recorded detailed field notes in which I described students' presences in class and noted, for instance, aspects of their physical appearance, such as skin color and how they dressed and wore their hair. I also listed material artifacts they brought to class, such as coffee mugs, notebooks, backpacks, essay drafts, skateboards, and planners, because I noticed these things as mattering to the interactional scenes I was observing. As I worked with the recordings of students' classroom conversations, however, I very early on realized that I had to be exceptionally careful in making connections between the observations recorded in my field notes and what students themselves might be apprehending or orienting to. One way to make such links was to notice when students commented on or indexed them in talk. Given the depth of what is potentially available for perception and the shallowness of what is consciously attended (which I discuss in chapter 1), such explicit commentary entails only a fragment of what is influencing or motivating students' interactional behaviors and classroom utterances. This presented an important analytic challenge. While I was certain that clothing and other material accoutrements played active roles in students' identity performances and social negotiations, both my emphasis on marking difference through talk and interaction and the time frame of the data generation (one semester) constrained what questions I could answer about students' perceptions of their own and others' presences, the environmental surround, and material artifacts.

After completing *Toward a New Rhetoric of Difference*, I continued to wrestle with what still felt undone or unsettled in this work. To do this, I spent time thinking about difference as it worked in my own life, which meant considering race and gender but also disability and, significantly later, deafness, as particularly important differences for attention and study. I reflected on my own choice making around clothing, hair, physical appearance, and whiteness. I noticed my reactions to various physical and virtual environments. I attended to shifts in ongoing relationships in my workplace and in my personal life. I paid special attention to how whiteness operated in my actions and perceptions as well as how racism, misogyny, and gender-based discrimination functioned in my interactions with others. These reflections influenced my turn to questions about disability disclosure in academic scholarship[44] and about how writing scholars accounted for disability in classroom anecdotes.[45] I was interested in not only how disability materialized as I interacted with other people but also how experiences of disability influenced interactional choices and rhetorical practices. To do this work, I needed to be able to account for the materiality of the world and of bodyminds moving in shared interactional space. Consequently, this book is a different kind of exploration than the one I performed in *Toward*.

In making a turn to disability as a line of inquiry, the methodology that I have taken centers on narrative. I have sought out all kinds of stories that people tell about experiences of disability. Through lived experiences, we build our perceptual practices, and these practices are differently attuned to disability. These different perceptual apparatuses are also differently attuned to disability's imbrication and co-constitution within interlocking systems of oppression. In this way, the stories we tell of disability are shaped by every aspect of our embodied materiality that comes to be perceived and made available for noticing within systems of power and valuation. These commitments have helped me cultivate an orientation to disability in my daily movements and interactions, and they have motivated several forms of narrative data generation. I have collected images of signs that called disability to my attention. In this collecting, I have kept track of the stories that I and others have told about these signs. I have also assembled written accounts that might point to disability, even and perhaps especially when those texts might not be identified from the outset as being about disability. Additional stories emerged through a collaborative interview study that generated thirty-three narrative-based interviews with disabled faculty members. During these interviews, interviewees shared accounts of their experiences disclosing (or not disclosing) their disability in professional contexts. Alongside this narrative data set, I have been telling and writing and revising my own stories as I continue to shape my perceptual apparatus and practices of materializing disability. This book is an exploration of the everyday mattering and emergence of disability as well as disability's constitution in textual forms as a consequence of this mattering. The life I have lived is as much a component of this book as is my academic thinking and professional labor, and there is so much more yet to be explored.

1

Dis-Attending

Signs of disability emerge and take shape as observational apparatuses—what I will call from here on "perceptual apparatuses," building on Karen Barad's framework of agential realism—intra-act with the world's materiality and enact agential cuts that put boundaries around a phenomenon and link it to disability. Such materializations occur within environmental surrounds that shape what and how agential cuts are enacted. This chapter considers how perceptual practices to which many people are enculturated participate in disability's materialization. I use the term "*dis*-attention" to describe these perceptual practices, distinguishing between dominant *dis*-attentions that are taught and learned through often unattended details of everyday experience and disabled *dis*-attentions by which disabled people, through everyday lived experience, learn to perceive differently. Before I offer a definition and theoretical explanation of "*dis*-attention," however, let me start with a story.

I wrote and researched significant chunks of this book during 2019–2020 in a scholar-in-residence position at the National Center for Institutional Diversity (NCID), a research center at the University of Michigan. Being on a new campus and meeting all kinds of new colleagues was an exhilarating experience full of intellectual energy and generative discoveries for this extrovert as I navigated between the NCID suite, the U-M libraries, and my writing space in the English Department. However, despite the joy I experienced as I researched and wrote and engaged with intellectual and activist communities across the Michigan campus, spending an academic year at the University of Michigan was also incredibly demoralizing because of my experience with faculty accommodation. When NCID offered me the scholar-in-residence opportunity, they made clear their expectation that scholars would be in residence and engaged in campus life while pursuing their research. Given what I know about the work it takes for participation in academic life to be meaningful for me (see introduction), I opened a conversation about accommodations.

I was stunned to learn that there is no university-wide process at Michigan for faculty accommodation. The policy in the College of Literature, Science, and Arts (LSA) is, essentially, that a disabled employee should negotiate any accommodations they need with their supervisor.[1] For me, this meant negotiating directly with NCID, a small research center on campus, putting primary responsibility for covering the cost of my interpreting needs on their budget as well as expecting their staff to perform the labor of identifying and securing interpreters and captioners for their events. No one at the center had any previous experience with sign language interpreting or real-time captioning, and so our conversations about this started at the beginning, with everyone involved working to learn as much as they could as quickly as possible. This was a lot. As Teresa Blankmeyer Burke notes in her work on sign language interpreting ethics, making communication-access arrangements in academic contexts is far from a simple or straightforward task and involves highly specialized knowledge and the cultivation of ongoing, long-term relationships with both deaf academics and access providers.[2] Indeed, it was incredibly difficult to procure reliable, high-quality communication access during my time at Michigan. This was a complicated situation influenced by high demand for access provision and a low supply of providers; my newness to the community and lack of personal connections; and a general paucity of knowledge around access provision at the university. But it was also tightly tied to the LSA expectation that sponsoring units and departments were responsible for ensuring their events' accessibility and that there was no centralized space for consolidating and promoting what disability scholar and design theorist Aimi Hamraie has called "access knowledge" across the U-M campus.

Let me put this situation in a broader context. I note in the introduction to this book that my thinking about and relationships to disability have been shifting over a long period of time. I have now been living and working in large, predominantly white, public universities for more than twenty-five years, from my time as an undergrad at The Ohio State University through my graduate work at the University of Wisconsin–Madison to my experience as a faculty member at Texas A&M University, the University of Delaware, and, now, the University of Washington.

I have given talks and workshops for which I have made accommodation requests at more than twenty-five other institutions. I have also spent a lot of time, because of my research and scholarly expertise, talking to faculty about their accommodation experiences. And what I witnessed at Michigan is one of the most egregious situations that I have personally experienced. Yet, this situation in which faculty accommodation is treated as an afterthought is endemic in higher education, and has inequitable impacts on multiply minoritized disabled faculty.[3] What I name and theorize here as *dis*-attention is not particular to Michigan but is instead built in the accommodation process for most disabled faculty at colleges and universities across the United States.

In *Academic Ableism*, Jay Dolmage shows that higher education has from its beginnings again and again sought to set itself apart from disability, relegating disability to other spaces and educational environments.[4] Shunting disability to "special" times and places—which happened repeatedly during my scholar-in-residence experience as I ultimately made choices to selectively attend events according to the signs of disability I perceived—contributes to the challenge of noticing disability on campus. This difficulty of foregrounding disability is amplified by the disciplinary formation of disability studies and its recognizable institutionalized forms. Early disability studies work predominantly featured white disability studies scholars studying populations of white disabled people with physical disabilities, a phenomenon noted by Christopher Bell in his 2006 essay "Introducing White Disability Studies: A Modest Proposal," published in the second edition of the *Disability Studies Reader*.[5] Much has shifted in the sixteen years since Bell's essay was published, with scholars across an interdisciplinary range turning to sites and areas of study that decenter whiteness and approach disability not in representational terms as an identity or identification but as part of an interlocking system of relationships to power and sociality.[6] In an essay forwarding "feminist-of-color disability studies," Sami Schalk and Jina B. Kim emphasize the need for an understanding of disability that moves away from white-dominated frames, whether this refers to scholars' theoretical and citational apparatuses or the particular areas they study. Consequently, what is recognized as "disability" must be understood as inflected by other dominant and normative valuations of bodies within complex systems of power and domination.[7]

The concept of *dis*-attention builds on the backdrop of absence and erasure created by dominant and normative contexts, critiquing what gets elided and ignored when white-dominated scholarship and arenas of study forward particular understandings of disability. It also critiques the ways that many institutional environments—like Michigan's—actively forward and even depend on maintaining cultures of whiteness, in turn obscuring many ways that disability is always present as well as the ways that race, gender, sexuality, and citizenship intertwine to shape how disability materializes and comes to be perceived. To orient ourselves differently to disability and recognize the centrality of race to signs of disability, it may be useful to take up Sara Ahmed's discussion of disorientation. If, as she writes, whiteness is "a social and bodily orientation given that some bodies will be more at home in a world that is orientated around whiteness," then these orientations—e.g., "being at home" or "unstressed" around a body or in a place—will shape what becomes available for noticing as disability.[8] At Michigan, an institutional culture of whiteness serves to reinforce practices of *dis*-attention that elide disability and race. Institutional eliteness seeps from every nook and cranny of the U-M campus. For instance, the phrase "The Leaders and Best," a line from the university's fight song, echoes across campus in slogans, large flags and banners adorning buildings, invitations to join clubs and activities, and flyers plastered on nearly every vertical surface. This messaging feeds a culture that is replete with expectations of hyperproductivity and perfectionism and that contributes to the challenge of making disability available for noticing among U-M faculty. Outside of disability-focused spaces and communities at U-M, I experienced intense resistance to acknowledging that disabled people were part of the campus community, much less to being open to identifications with disability.

To orient differently, to *dis*-orient, I suggest we can practice *dis*-attention. *Dis*-attention is an intentionally awkward and clunky polyvalent neologism that I have coined to point to the many ways that disability, always entangled with race, gender, sexuality, and citizenship, is attended in everyday movements in the world. Perhaps the most prevalent forms of *dis*-attention involve singling disability out as a special or exceptional circumstance while simultaneously ignoring its everyday occurrences, such as treating questions of access as only for special bodies rather than as also part of the everyday life of the university. It also calls out the erasures that happen when experiences specific to particular populations—such as those of white, physically disabled people—are treated as if they represent disability experiences generally. This simultaneous emphasis and erasure is represented in "*dis*-attention" by separating the prefix "*dis*" with a hyphen as well as italicizing it. The point is to stress the compartmentalization of disability to "special" places, beings, and/or times while also playing on the meaning of the prefix "dis" as "removal, aversion, negation, reversal of action."[9]

The challenge of perceiving disability has been remarked by numerous scholars who acknowledge the everydayness of disability while critiquing its frequent elision or erasure. Many disability studies researchers have documented how disability is simultaneously articulated and elided within the specificity of particular historical, social, and material configurations. For instance, in Jaipreet Virdi's work curating an "Objects of Disability" archive, which collects and tracks disability artifacts across Canadian museums, she has confronted the challenge that disability is rarely catalogued by museum curators, and when it is, it is often as a medical artifact.[10] The consequence is that the everydayness of disability is largely ignored and the parameters shaping what a museum archives and indexes with a disability-findable tag is narrow. Prostheses, wheelchairs, mobility aids, and hearing aids and instruments are well represented in Virdi's catalog, while ramps, for instance (to take an example from Bess Williamson's work in *Accessible America*),[11] are not. But much like disability itself, *dis*-attention resists containment and often insists on escaping the boundaries placed around it.

One way that *dis*-attention slips away from concrete definition is in its invocation of attentions performed and enacted by disabled people and emerging out of disabled experiences. Take, for instance, my discussion in this book's introduction of how deafness is perceptible in all kinds of ways. I have learned to notice signs of deafness over time, through my lived experience as a white deaf woman in company at different times and places with other deaf people. I pay attention—*dis*-attend—differently as a consequence of the experiences I have had with my body and mind moving among material environments with all kinds of beings. *Dis*-attention as a polyvalent concept thus involves both dominant practices of simultaneous hyperperceptibility and erasure and disabled practices of attending that materialize different phenomena and enact different boundaries around these phenomena. Perception is always shifting over time and across contexts, attuning to some details while backgrounding and eliding others as we develop particular kinds of expertise and navigate different degrees of familiarity with particular kinds of encounters. There is much still to learn and understand about our perceptual practices because of the ways that dominant *dis*-attentions—including an overemphasis on visual modes of perception and the circulation of ableist narratives about disability—shape them. These dominant *dis*-attentions entangle with disabled forms of *dis*-attention to create new patterns and practices of perception.

Waves of *dis*-attention intra-act in encounters involving agents with different orientations to disability and who perform perception in different ways. Different ways of perceiving disability can interfere with or amplify one another. Disabled people often play on and resist dominant *dis*-attentions, sometimes by deflecting or avoiding attention to disability, such as by pointing to particular phenomena to deflect attention from other potentially perceptible phenomena. At other times, disability may be highlighted or explicitly signaled in order to encourage others to share in or take up new behaviors, practices, and orientations. In all of this, disability is inextricably imbricated with the full range of identifications that people perform and orient to in their daily lives and that emerge in complex constellations. For instance, hands moving in sign language might materialize deafness or disability on white bodies but, in another scene, materialize violence or aggression on Black and brown bodies, depending on the perceiver and other intra-acting phenomena in the environmental surround. This is not simply a hypothetical example conjured up for illustration here: example after example of documented violence against Black and brown people have become regular appearances on social media and news channels in recent years and underscore the ways that disability never appears alone.

With *dis*-attention I also want to underscore that sensory input of all kinds participates in the work of perceiving. Many discussions of sensory input build their theorizing upon assumptions of normative ranges of that sensory perception, obscuring differential forms of sensory attunement (*dis*-attentions) that disabled people develop,[12] as well as the ways that sensory perceptions are often multiple and interrelated. The ways that I perceive sound and make meaning from it, for instance, are rarely substantively accounted for in research on sound studies. In recent years there has been a growing attention to the valences of multisensory perception,[13] work that can usefully inform a more robust understanding of how sensory perception makes disability available for noticing, attention, and emergence.

I am always learning and coming-to-know my own practices of *dis*-attention, and I am influenced by the *dis*-attentions I have learned over the course of living a life as a white deaf woman. I am always building new relations and new orientations to disability. This means learning with others—both animate and inanimate—how each of our differential attunements[14] orient all of us in (different) ways and shape how we collectively and individually *dis*-attend. Coming to better understand the relationships and influences among the dominant and disabled *dis*-attentions that circulate around us is an essential part of learning to attend to disability. In many cases, because of the pervasive influence of dominant forms of *dis*-attention, we may need to learn to perceive disability differently, always in dynamic relation with our lived experiences and with the forms of perception to which we are continually encultured. This does not mean learning to perceive disabled bodyminds, as disability matters far beyond identity. It operates at an ideological level, such as through the "ideologies of ability" Tobin Siebers describes that uphold and affirm normativity and abled-ness,[15] as well as through various forms of biopower that determine what bodies can even have access to disability, as Jasbir Puar suggests in *The Right to Maim*.[16] Mel Chen's exploration of animacy—qualities of liveness or sentience attached to words or beings—further implicates disability, race, and queerness as historically specific and interrelated means of organizing bodies and minds and structuring social relations.[17] We cannot *only* attend to disability in and on particular bodies and minds.

With *dis*-attention, then, my aim is to invite attention not simply to disability's emergence as a way of identifying or categorizing people but also to its ongoing function as a shaping and structuring concept that matters in the world's becoming. Indeed, as Michael Bérubé, Maren Linett, Julia Miele Rodas, and Rebecca Sanchez have each shown in their analyses of embodied authorship, textual arrangement, and narrative coherence, texts themselves can be disabled; disability can be invoked abstractly, without attaching to a body or object at all; and myriad configurations can invite or close off attention to disability.[18] I hope to encourage attention to the perceptual practices that lead us to notice disability or, more commonly, not-notice it. These perceptual practices are at work shaping and reshaping dominant and disabled forms of *dis*-attention in even the most mundane of encounters.

Let us come back to Michigan and my experiences of navigating faculty accommodations to illustrate how signs of disability are taken up by disabled and dominant practices of *dis*-attention. Once again, it is important to acknowledge that Michigan is an egregious—but not singular—example here. The college's policy for faculty accommodation, which pointed disabled faculty to their supervisors to negotiate for accommodations that they might need, and which put the onus for access provision on the unit or entity hosting an event, meant that I was negotiating not only with NCID regarding my responsibilities as a member of the center's community but also with every single unit or group who was sponsoring an event I wanted to be part of. That is, if I wanted to attend a talk hosted by the Department of American Studies, say, or if the English Department asked me to be on a panel, those departments were responsible for the event's accessibility and accommodation. This created a paradoxical situation of *dis*-attention in which everyone was responsible for access and accommodation, which in practice meant nobody was responsible.

Ironically enough, given the fact that cost has dominated many of my interactions around access and accommodation over the last two decades, at Michigan, money was never the issue. Everyone was willing to pay, and no one ever gave me grief about how much communication access cost.[19] NCID faculty and staff members were unfailingly kind and ready to do what was needed to ensure my accommodations. But no matter how nice they were about it, I was still aware that my accommodations cost them significant time, effort, and money. The center's leadership and staff worked across Michigan's sprawling and highly decentralized structure to identify pockets of disability-accommodation knowledge or experience that they could build on, and they curated a Google spreadsheet of local sign language interpreters, agencies, and real-time captioning providers that they made available to anyone at U-M needing to secure interpreting or captioning.[20] They did find some institutional resources and support funds, but most were earmarked for specific kinds of structural access (e.g., installing a ramp, widening a door, or putting up a flashing smoke alarm) rather than for the ongoing communication access I needed.

In many ways, NCID was in the situation of needing to reinvent an already-invented-many-times-over wheel. The Americans with Disabilities Act, the law that mandates reasonable accommodation in workplaces across the United States, was passed in 1990. People had been developing practices and infrastructures supporting accommodation provision in higher education for more than thirty years, and effective practices existed at many of U-M's peer institutions, including The Ohio State University, thanks to L. Scott Lissner's leadership, which I often pointed to during my time at Michigan as a positive example. (I sometimes think about how lucky it was that I fell in love with Ohio State and didn't consider going to college anywhere else, because such provision was already—when I arrived on campus in 1995—part of the institutional fabric and mediated by my access to whiteness. I didn't have to fight for it; it was offered and encouraged, and that has made all the difference.)[21] Amidst this environment of *dis*-attention, it did not take long for me to get clear with myself that my highest priority was focusing on my academic scholarship during my sabbatical and that I could not give over my scholar-in-residence period to the work of changing faculty accommodation procedures at the University of Michigan. This led me to decide early on that I would only selectively attend events, prioritizing those that would be most important or helpful to the work I was doing as well as—as I had done in learning to navigate professional conferences early in my career—those that signaled their attention to disability and access.

I got excited when emails started arriving in my Michigan email inbox about Disability Community Month events. Disability Community Month, I learned, had previously been called "Investing in Ability," at least up until the late 1990s,[22] but its name was changed after lobbying from the Council for Disability Concerns (CfDC), a loosely organized coalition of disabled faculty and staff with access to extremely modest institutional funding, who protested the event's emphasis on "ability," noting that the title centered nondisabled perspectives, ignored the contributions and importance of the disability community, and did little to encourage substantive change in culture, behaviors, and practices at U-M. I had been invited to participate on a panel titled "An Ingenious

Way to Live: Fostering Disability Culture in Higher Education," and conversations about that event had centered access considerations, including explicit reminders to write into our scripts physical descriptions of ourselves and to ensure that all the panelists coordinated around different access moves.

This backdrop informed my decision to request accommodations for two events advertised on a flyer for several Disability Community Month events circulated through the CfDC listserv. Given the signs of disability I had already encountered, not just in the planning around "An Ingenious Way to Live" but also through interactions with CfDC members, involvement on a university-wide task force charged with reporting on and making recommendations for disability at U-M, and connections with faculty involved with disability studies on campus, the events featured on this flyer seemed like ones I should make an effort to attend. They also felt like opportunities to connect with other disability-interested colleagues across campus. But red flags—signs of dominant *dis*-attention that tend to subsume the particularities of specific disability experiences and ignore the complexities of access—came up quickly. The first one was that the flyer did not have any information about whom to contact to make accommodation requests, nor did it communicate what accessibility features were already incorporated into the events it was advertising. Taking a deep breath, I looked at who had sent the original email. While the flyer had circulated on the CfDC listserv, the return address for the original mailing was a generic "Disability@UMich.Edu" address—another sign of dominant *dis*-attention. While generic addresses like this one can be useful for ensuring that a group or organization's communication is not solely one person's responsibility, I have also found that I cannot assume that people who monitor such accounts have any idea how to navigate accommodation and access requests. The responses I have gotten when making this kind of outreach have ranged wildly.

So, I wrote, not sure what to expect and having no idea where the email would go, the following email:

> Dear Disability@UMich.Edu,
> I don't quite know to whom this email goes, but I would like to request sign language interpreting for a few of the upcoming Disability

Community Month Events. I am cc'ing —— at NCID who has been building a list of interpreting agencies and contacts and may be able to share that list with you if you need any additional information or leads. I'm also attaching to this email a letter that I ask be shared with any interpreter(s) working with me so that they can prepare adequately and ensure their readiness to meet my particular interpreting needs.

Below are the events that I've tentatively put on my calendar, pending interpreting availability. In addition, could the speaker(s) be asked to provide access copies of any scripts they are working from? This helps me follow along, and also goes a long way to support interpreting access.

Despite not knowing what to expect, I really was not prepared for the deluge of emails that ensued. I witnessed the real-time unfolding of many people doing their best to figure out how they could secure interpreting or captioning for two Disability Community Month events, in a seemingly endless chain of "do you know . . ."; "can you . . ."; and exchanges of small bits of information and knowledge from one person to another that underscored that no one was building access knowledge[23] around sign language interpreting and accommodation to any significant degree anywhere on Michigan's main campus where I was living and working.

To put this another way, there is an entire institutional practice and history of *dis*-attention at U-M that put the onus for accommodation on individual disabled faculty to spend their time negotiating accommodations repeatedly and unceasingly again and again and again and again. Annika Konrad has theorized this incessant demand as "access fatigue," describing it as "the everyday pattern of constantly needing to help others participate in access, a demand so taxing that it can accumulate to the point of giving up on access altogether," a concept that builds on theorizing around racial microaggressions.[24] Access fatigue is prevalent in higher education, where institutional cultures, policies, and practices relentlessly *dis*-attend—elide and ignore the everydayness of disability. Such conditions set any disabled individual seeking to enact change up for failure. In many ways, I am grateful that this all unfolded in my second month at Michigan, because it illustrated the depths of dominant *dis*-attention across the campus and solidified my resolve to aggressively conserve my energy around networking and trying to attend events.

I had already learned from my previous experiences negotiating structures for accommodation how much time and energy this work took, and I put up significant boundaries around the time and energy I was willing to give over to it at U-M. That I was on sabbatical was really the only thing that made the tenuousness of my accommodations and the relentlessness of needing to explain my access needs again and again not a source of extraordinary stress. If I did not receive accommodations for a meeting or an event, I could shrug and say, "Well, that's more time to focus on writing my book," and go on about my day. If I did not feel as though I could muster the energy for one more access conversation, the consequences were relatively minor: my disappointment, my exclusion from the event, and the loss of opportunity for others to interact with me. My ability to shrug at this situation, however, was supported by significant privileges I experience—of whiteness, of tenure, and of my transitory status on campus. In situations of permanent or precarious employment, intersectional oppressions, or institutional transition, the stakes of these kinds of everyday exclusion are exponentially higher. Ultimately, because I did not have reliable access to high-quality sign language interpreting or computer-aided real-time translation (CART) transcription—a structural reality shaped by myriad, embedded, and deeply rooted dominant *dis*-attentions that infused every space, environment, and interaction on the U-M campus—the conditions for building any kind of relationships, the resonances that I could amplify, the associations I could try to mobilize and amplify, were limited.

My individual experience was subsumed by waves of *dis*-attentions that constrained possibilities. I found myself again and again exerting efforts to make disability available for those around me to perceive. Everyone knew that I was deaf, but they had no idea what that meant, or what they should do, so I had to explain every time I wanted to attend something. This is by no means specific to Michigan; it has always been part of my life. I have always had to negotiate between the signs of disability that others readily identify, the signs that I purposefully display or call attention to, and those that are available within my environment for both conscious and nonconscious perception that shape what people noticed about me. Any time I made decisions about whether to attend an event or even ask after accommodations, I sought out signs of disability that might indicate an awareness of the need for accessibility or the elision entirely of accessibility considerations. I learned to perceive in my disabled way an environment's or interaction's potential accessibility or hospitality. Building disabled *dis*-attentions enabled me to navigate interactional encounters and persist in various institutional environments. The signs of disability that I sought out as well as those that I actively displayed in navigating my time at Michigan were always consequential, always taking shape as the result of interactions among dominant and disabled *dis*-attentions of all kinds.

My hope with this book is to encourage some ways for us to cultivate perceptual apparatuses attuned to the signs of disability all around us as we experience the entanglement of matter and meaning. Learning to notice practices of *dis*-attention is one way to productively move toward such activity. In the remainder of this chapter, then, I explain why it is often incredibly challenging—but also exceptionally urgent—to participate in a process of intentionally reshaping our perceptual apparatuses. I first discuss Therí Pickens's intersectional materialist approach to reading the folds of Blackness and madness alongside Barad's framework of agential realism to emphasize how intra-actions between perceptual apparatus and material reality give (some) definition to signs of disability. I then take up a set of material signs I encountered in my time at Michigan to show how Asia Friedman's sociological exploration of gender perception and perceptual filtering further extends our understanding of *dis*-attention. Finally, pulling together the threads of multisensory perception, perceptual apparatuses, perceptual filtering, and disabled forms of *dis*-attention, I read two signs of disability—my hearing aids and a closed caption logo—to suggest how a signs-of-disability analysis might proceed.

Agential Realism and Perceptual Apparatuses

Dis-attention is both an orientation and a practice, and like any practice, it can be learned and cultivated. Many of us have been enculturated to not-notice disability, to avoid it and keep it at arm's length. I am reminded of this on a regular basis through habitual encounters, from others' frequent descriptions of me as "hearing impaired" (a term I do not use to describe myself) to awkward negotiations when my use of "disability" is corrected to "ability" to the fact that I am regularly informed that I should always use person-first language. Each of these examples reinforces the challenge of making disability perceptible to others, especially in environments where people are motivated to hide, minimize, or suppress disability's presence.

What does it mean to perceive disability? Barad's agential realist framework responds to this question by suggesting perception as a material-discursive practice that enacts boundaries and gives definition to properties of observed phenomena. The materiality of perception involves bodily apparatuses—nerves, receptors, and neural fibers—that communicate sensory input to the brain as well as the ways that the world's materiality becomes available for perception. Sometimes this availability comes through shared, synchronous copresence in physical space, but it just as often happens at geographical and/or temporal removes. We tell stories, for instance. We peruse photographs and watch videos. We read books and essays. All of these things are material and become available to us through various apparatuses such as fiber optic Internet cables, screen readers, paper and glue, tablets and computers, digital files, metadata, and Braille interfaces. In Barad's terms, whether we are using an electron tunneling microscope to observe particles at the quantum level or using our embodied materiality to move sensory perceptions of human interaction into (un)conscious awareness, our body-minds and our means of sensory perception are themselves intra-acting with particular configurations of the world to materialize phenomena. Barad uses the clunky and unintuitive term "intra-action" rather than "interaction" to emphasize "that distinct agencies do not precede, but rather emerge through, their intra-action."[25]

A second answer to the question of how disability comes to be perceived is forwarded in Pickens's materialist and intersectional theorizing as she reads Blackness and madness together. As Pickens writes, "Material reality must reckon with what others have pointed out are the lived experiences of the Black and disabled body, what amount to (in this project, at least) the gaps and folds within Black speculative fiction." Such a reading, she argues, must grapple with "concerns at the heart of disability studies: pain, fiscal access, and the validity of embodied experience."[26] Of particular importance here is Pickens's critique of mutual constitution as a reading strategy, one that resonates alongside Barad's discussion of Neils Bohr's concept of indeterminacy. In discussing mutual constitution, Pickens notes that while the phrase might imply a "reciprocity of creation," that reciprocity—"simultaneity while occupying the temporal plane"—is rarely realized for both terms in the equation. She further challenges the assumption that many "discourses and material conditions related to race and disability . . . develop and are sustained completely and consistently."[27] For instance, meanings associated with disability and race frequently lead to Blackness and madness being cast in the service of resisting ableism and reinforcing preexisting narrative frames rather than being attended to in order to materialize alternative boundaries and phenomena. "Thinking through the Black mad subject," Pickens writes, "we must consider that this person is meant not only to occupy space but to be consistently removed from space in order to make room for the more recognizable subject: the white able body."[28] Pickens's theorizing stresses the challenge of realizing mutuality or constitution amidst environments and practices of storying that consistently erase Blackness and disability and (re)center whiteness and ability.

We can also come to understand some of the challenges for realizing mutuality and constitution through Barad's discussion of Bohr's work on indeterminacy. Bohr's concept of indeterminacy says that complementary phenomena are not simultaneously determinate—that is, they do not simultaneously have definition. While Bohr's definition of indeterminacy is sometimes conflated with Heisenberg's uncertainty principle, which states that multiple components of an equation are not simultaneously knowable, Bohr is making an ontic claim while Heisenberg's is epistemic. Barad explains: Heisenberg's uncertainty principle "favors the notion that measurements disturb existing values, thereby placing a limit on our knowledge of the situation."[29] In other words, the classical paradigm assumes that when we perceive one or more dimensions of a phenomenon, the other dimensions are still out there and we just do not know what they are. In contrast, Bohr's formulation asserts that "properties are only determinate given the existence of particular material arrangements that give definition to the corresponding concept in question. In the absence of such conditions, the corresponding properties do not have determinate values."[30]

If, as Bohr argues, matter does not have determinate properties until it is observed, then its properties are indeterminate until they are measured. It is not that certain properties are unknown, in other words; it is that a particular configuration has not materialized them yet—they do not exist until they materialize. Within Bohr's model, perceptual apparatuses intra-act with the matter being observed and produce a phenomenon. It is this phenomenon that is ultimately perceived, not matter in and of itself, and the emergence of a phenomenon involves the enactment of an agential cut that makes determinate some, but not all, properties of the phenomenon. Measurement, then, "is an instance where matter and meaning meet in a literal sense."[31]

The stories we tell reveal the phenomena we perceive. Pickens's work helps us understand this as she confronts the challenges inherent in observation and narrative. Her response is to insist on "contextualiz[ing] madness in communities of Blackness rather than in exclusive relation to a white cisheteropatriarchal norm."[32] This move resonates with Barad's reminder that there is no outside from which the world can be observed and documented; any observation is itself an intra-action, an involvement, a being *of* the world in which observers participate in and shape the very phenomena they are perceiving. What passes through perceptual apparatuses, Pickens and Barad each remind us, is not reality but the outcomes of specific configurations of material-discursive practices that shape emergent phenomena.

An example that Barad shares may help further illustrate these intra-actions between perceptual apparatuses and phenomena. One scientific problem that quantum physics has helped resolve involves what is sometimes colloquially referred to as the "wave-particle duality" of light, which acknowledges that light behaves and has properties of both particles and waves. Grounded in a classical (that is, not quantum) approach, the wave-particle duality assumed matter's stability and took as its goal that of building better, and more precise, observational apparatuses in order to get at better understandings of the natural world. However, quantum approaches challenge the idea that matter has determinate properties that human observers can identify and name. Bohr's indeterminacy principle recognizes matter's indeterminacy by acknowledging the intra-action between measuring apparatus and observed entity. In other words, how we observe shapes what is observed. It is the intra-action between the measuring apparatus and light that leads to its materialization, making determinate either motion or position but not both.[33] To return to Pickens, then, the method and practice of observing, of moving among the folds of Blackness and madness, that she performs is itself essential to coming to realize "how the discourses of madness and Blackness not only operate in intraracial intimate spaces but also intensify and dismantle common understandings of each other."[34] Our knowledge-making practices, the means by which we observe reality, involve intra-actions between perceptual apparatuses and objects of observation that ultimately determine—put boundaries around—some properties of the phenomena we perceive.

Together, Pickens and Barad support a model of disability perceptibility that underscores disability as emerging when a perceptual apparatus intra-acts with sensory input to give definition to some properties of a phenomenon, linking it to disability in some way. As we live and move and experience with particular bodies and minds in dynamic relations with the world, those experiences are always participating in intra-actions producing perceived phenomena. How these phenomena are interpreted is "the effect of boundary-drawing practices that make some identities or attributes intelligible (determinate) to the exclusion of others."[35] Different agential cuts reveal different properties. In this way, "knowledge-making practices" are "material enactments that contribute to, and are part of, the phenomena we describe."[36] This is not to say that perceptual apparatuses create phenomena. One person declaring "disability!" will not necessarily, for others, adhere meaningfully to a phenomenon, and material-discursive practices are always intra-acting, often in ways outside of direct awareness or consciousness. We can use this framework to ask what it means to "count" as a deaf person. When I am around hearing people who have little to no experience with deaf people, my deafness materializes—matters—in different ways than it does when I am interacting with someone who claims significant experience with deaf people, whether personally or professionally or both. Every intra-action I experience differentially enacts boundaries and makes determinate different properties associated with deafness. And these properties and boundaries are not just about deafness as a singular category but are always coalescing and materializing in entangled relationships with all the other identifications that matter to perceptions of intra-acting phenomena.

Categories such as disability, race, gender, class, nationality, and sexuality, then, are not simply socially constructed terms that shape how people understand and organize themselves but are themselves emergent phenomena taking shape as a result of intra-actions among material bodies, observational (measuring) apparatuses, and their iterative working and reworking. Understanding categories in this way links reality—phenomena that materialize through intra-actions between perceptual apparatuses and the world—with myriad other emerging and intra-acting phenomena, in which categories "materialize through, and are enfolded into, one another."[37] Such topological shifts and dynamics again resonate with Pickens's reading of constellations between Blackness and madness that recognizes that "in Black cultural and critical contexts, disability is often operating in other registers."[38] Pickens further notes that traditional reading practices frame race and disability as competing for focus. Pickens insists on refusing essentialist fixations on single identity categories that linger in cultural imaginations and continue to inflect even those reading practices aimed at engaging multiple identifications. Michael Hames-García forwards "identity multiplicity" as a potentially useful means of attending to identity categories as blending and shifting, much as shades of only three colors—yellow, blue, and red—make up every photograph, but nevertheless enable extraordinary diversity and complexity.[39]

Again, while it is common to think of multiple identities as mutually constituting—influencing—one another, we do not yet, as Pickens argues, have a strong theory for how such mutual influence might occur nor for interpreting their dynamic and emergent possibilities. David Valentine points to this problem of identity multiplicity and perceptual emergence as he questions the influence that academic classifications have on how bodies are figured. In his survey of anthropological literature pulled under a transgender studies umbrella, Valentine shows that rather than forwarding a cohesive notion of a "transgender" category, these texts reveal instead that "age, race, class, and so on don't merely inflect or intersect with those experiences we call gender and sexuality but rather *shift the very boundaries of what 'gender' and 'sexuality' can mean* in particular contexts."[40] In other words, identity multiplicity involves the entanglement of matter and meaning that leads to the production of phenomena that beings can perceive and process as sensory input.

Each of the interpersonal encounters Valentine recounts in his book involves various forms of physical and virtual copresence in which people's bodily materiality is perceived in various ways. These encounters create sensory input that passes through and intra-acts with participants' perceptual apparatuses and participates in new intra-acting phenomena. Identity categories, such as deafness or transgender, then, are not simply produced in individuals in predictable formulations; they involve complex intra-acting phenomena that themselves complexly intra-act and lead to different emergent phenomena. Categories into which people might organize themselves and others are always being revised and their boundaries reconstituted through dynamic material-discursive configurations and intra-actions. The messiness of transgender as a category that Valentine identifies is not only because of the complexity of identity labels and shifting identifications but also because of the intra-acting agencies of material forms of embodiment and copresence in shared virtual and physical spaces, all of which involve various interpersonal and textual means of making categories, relationships, and forms of perception available for others to apprehend.

Such processes of materializing social categories—textually and interactionally—have long been integral to a robust literature on passing,[41] masking,[42] and covering[43] and offer important sites for learning to perceive differently. One prominent example of this work is Ellen Samuels's now-canonical queer disability studies essay "My Body, My Closet," which works through the complex dynamics as well as the analogical limitations involved in reading across gender, sexuality, race, and disability. Samuels narrates her experiences of what she calls "nonvisible disability" (and which some now term "nonapparent disability") alongside those of how a femme gender category is frequently obscured within lesbian communities.[44] The erasures and ellipses that get enacted when identity categories compete for attention (precisely the issue Pickens lays out for mutual constitution) are pointedly illustrated in C. Riley Snorton's reading of race and gender as fungible categories in William and Ellen Craft's *Running a Thousand Miles for Freedom*. The Crafts' account is often treated as a narrative of gender and racial passing that describes how in 1848, Ellen Craft donned a gentleman's hat and clothing, as well as a poultice over her chin and a sling, to present as William Johnson, a traveling gentleman, while William Craft presented himself as Johnson's servant as they fled across the Atlantic to England. Snorton's analysis acknowledges that while "the logic of passing would apprehend Ellen's cross-gendered fugitivity as the primary case of gender fungibility," William Craft also participates in this gender fungibility in becoming a "disability 'prop'" that supports Ellen's transformation into Mr. Johnson. In this way, "the Crafts' narrative illustrates [that] fungibility and fugitivity figured two sides of a Janus-faced coin, in which the same logic that figured blackness as immanently interchangeable would also engender its flow."[45] The categorical interchangeability—fungibility—that Snorton brilliantly reveals throughout *Black on Both Sides* reinforces the stakes of shifting and changing perceptual practices and building new perceptual apparatuses. Such shifts in perceptual apparatus are part of Snorton's "attempt to find a vocabulary for black and trans life."[46]

Creating more livable—antiracist, anti-ableist—worlds is an essential project for higher education, which has a long history of exclusion that feeds a wide range of systemic inequities. The public land-grant institutions where I have lived and worked since 1995 originated from and continue to profit from wealth stolen from Indigenous land, as Robert Lee and Tristan Ahtone powerfully elaborate in "Land-Grab Universities."[47] This wealth has funded bastions of exclusivity, white supremacy, and inequity, all of which were on full display during my time at Michigan. Take, for instance, Angell Hall, the campus building where I spent most of my writing time. Angell is a large, imposing, five-story building featuring huge columns and steep steps that lead to the first-floor entrance. Steep steps are both a symbolic and material indicator of inaccessibility that Dolmage has theorized as literal and metaphorical means by which institutions make various forms of exclusion perceptible. "The self or selves that have been projected upon the space of the university," Dolmage writes, "are not just able-bodied and normal, but exceptional, *elite*. This projection unites many other discourses of normativity: whiteness, heteronormativity, empire, colonialism, masculinity."[48] This institutional eliteness, Dolmage shows, is essential to portraying higher education as a space and environment where disabled bodies and especially multiply marginalized, racially minoritized, queer, and trans disabled bodies are not expected or imagined. As Ahmed notes, "Spaces are orientated 'around' whiteness," and "the effect of this 'around whiteness' is the institutionalization of a certain 'likeness,' which makes nonwhite bodies uncomfortable and feel exposed, visible, and different when they take up this space."[49] Such imaginings shape not only the material encounter

between disabled bodies and inaccessible spaces but also the relationships, contestations, and coalitions that materialize all kinds of marginalized bodies and minds.

Collective Attention and Perceptual Filtering

I have yet to visit a college campus whose buildings are not difficult-
to-navigate labyrinthine spaces. The design and presence of directional
signage is often suggestive of the range of bodies and minds who might
be expected or behaviors that might be common within a particular
space. Are those moving through this space expected to be familiar with
it? Are they expected to need wayfinding support? Are there particular
spaces that often need to be navigated to, perhaps at particular times
of the year, as when brightly colored flyers might point to classroom
areas and then be removed once students have, presumably, familiarized
themselves with the building? In some ways, these directional signs can
be understood as retrofits, a second spatial metaphor for ableism that
Dolmage theorizes. Retrofitting refers to a process whereby something
that is inaccessible is made accessible after the fact, after it has already
been designed and revealed to be inaccessible for particular bodies and/
or minds. While retrofits are often interpreted as fixing a space's inaccessibility, Dolmage notes that they nevertheless "have a chronicity—a
timing and a time logic—that renders them highly temporary yet also
relatively unimportant."[50]

The after-the-fact addition as well as the temporariness and unim-
portance of the retrofit can be read in the photograph in figure 1.1,[51]
which features a yellow wall in Haven Hall, which is connected to Angell. You would encounter this wall when entering one of the primary
accessible entrances to Angell. The photograph shows three signs on the
wall. A pair of plastic maroon signs engraved in white offer building
directions. One sports an arrow pointing to the left, indicating how to
access classroom auditoriums and Tisch Hall; below it, a second sign has
a wheelchair icon at the top and the words "Elevator To Angell & Planetarium" and an arrow pointing straight ahead. A third sign is placed
just to the left of the two maroon ones. This one is made of paper and
has a thick yellow border on the left and bottom that features the words
"Orientation Michigan" in large blue letters. At the center is a white flyer

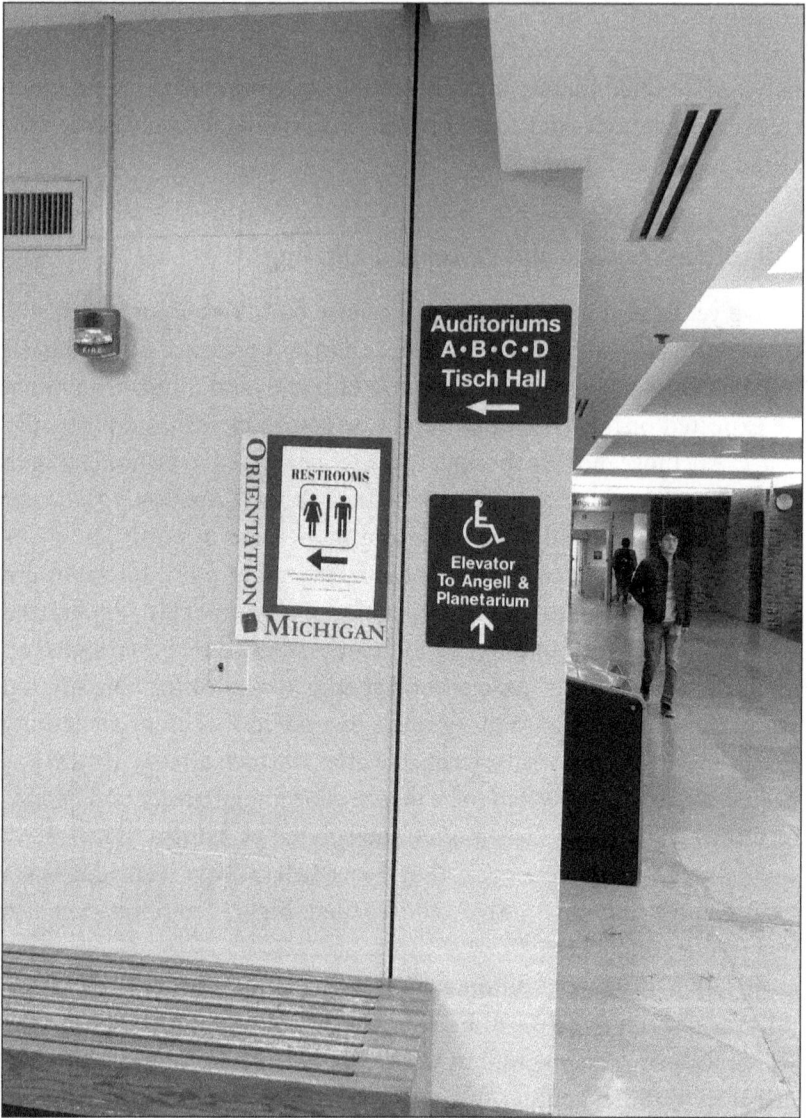

Figure 1.1. Directional Signage at the University of Michigan. Image description: A mustard-yellow wall sports two large maroon signs. One reads "Auditoriums A B C D Tisch Hall ←" and the other has a wheelchair logo on it, along with "Elevator to Angell and Planetarium" and an arrow pointing straight ahead. There is also a third sign just to the left of the two maroon ones. Made of paper, this sign has a thick yellow border on the left and bottom that features the words "Orientation Michigan" in large lettering. At the center is a white flyer with the word "Restrooms" in bold and all-caps. Just below "Restrooms" is a rectangle with two icons signaling male and female bodies separated with a bold line and an arrow pointing to the left. In smaller font that is not legible in the photo, this sign notes that a gender-inclusive bathroom is on the fifth floor of Angell Hall. The right edge of the photo shows the hallway leading to Angell; a recycling station lines the wall and a person in the distance is walking toward the camera. Ann Arbor, Michigan. (Photo by author.)

with the word "Restrooms" in bold and all-caps. Just below "Restrooms" is a rectangle with two binary-gendered figures separated with a bold line and an arrow pointing to the left. In a smaller font that is not legible in the photo, this sign notes that a gender-inclusive bathroom is on the fifth floor of Angell Hall.

I took this picture with my cell phone midway through the Fall 2019 semester as I was starting to get my bearings and figure out which entrances I could use to navigate to and from my office in Angell Hall. I have returned to this image often because it helps show how practices of *dis*-attention emerge from intra-actions between perceptual apparatuses and material reality. I took the picture to capture everyday signage that I passed on a daily basis. I noticed both the maroon signage and the paper sign pointing to the bathrooms, but I did not make any meaning of the "Orientation Michigan" border around the bathroom sign until much later. I also did not pay attention to the fine print on the bathroom signs beyond noting that the arrow pointed to the men's and women's restrooms while the text noted that the gender-inclusive bathroom was on the fifth floor (right by my office, in fact).

It was not until I was on the brink of leaving Michigan for good in Spring 2020 as the COVID-19 pandemic began to spread that I took a new perspective on these everyday spaces. Now, rather than orienting to them as part of the fabric of my daily existence, I was newly aware that I might never return to these buildings and was looking around anew. I was dumbfounded when I finally noticed the exceptionally small print on the bathroom signs that I had been moving past all year long that read "Facilities: Please save until August 3rd." Once I noticed that, I made a further connection between the signs' materiality and the "Orientation Michigan" border. Noticing both "August 3rd" and the border finally clued me in that these signs were probably placed for new-student orientation. Figure 1.2 shows a more readable view of that small print on a different sign placed next to the first-floor elevators in Angell. The sign is similar to the one in figure 1.1, with a few differences. Instead of two figures separated by a thick line, this sign shows only one figure,[52] its arrow points to the right, and its text reads, "Elevator to 5th floor gender inclusive restroom."

In March 2020 the signs were still up in various places with no indication that anyone was planning on replacing or removing them. The time

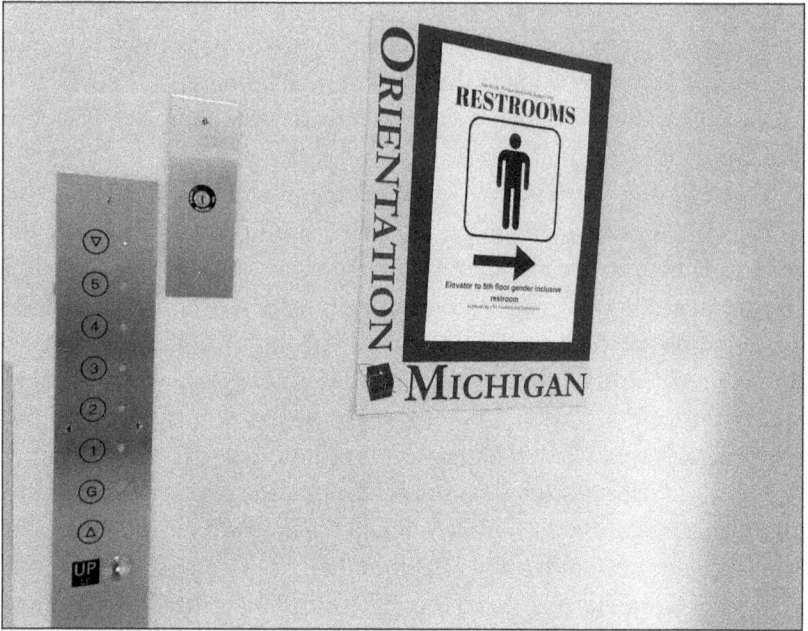

Figure 1.2. "Gender Inclusive Restroom" Sign by Angell Hall Elevator. Image Description: A restroom sign on a pale-yellow wall just to the right of an elevator panel. Made of paper, this sign has a thick yellow border on the left and bottom that features the words "Orientation Michigan" in large lettering. At the center is a white flyer with the word "Restrooms" in bold and all-caps. The differences between the sign in this photograph and the one above are that instead of two figures representing male and female separated by a thick line, here there is only one figure, and the bold but small-font text below the figure reads "Elevator to 5th floor gender inclusive restroom." Ann Arbor, Michigan. (Photo by author.)

logic and chronicity of these signs is tied to their materiality. That they are made of paper suggests their temporality, likely put up for a specific group of people (new students) and for a specific duration (until August 3rd). But if they were temporary, why were they not taken down? I can imagine multiple stories in response to these questions. One story is that the signs were put up and then forgotten. However, other details surrounding these signs challenge this story. For one thing, the signs are located near other directional signage and by elevators; for another, there were designated locations for flyers, advertisements, course listings, etc., and these were regularly cleared and maintained. Another, perhaps better story might be that after their utility at new-student orientation became apparent, the signs were intentionally left up. The fifth-floor gender-inclusive bathroom would be impossible for someone to find if they did not already know it was there. But here again, the visual and tactile differences between the plastic-engraved maroon signage and the large blue-and-yellow-and-white paper restroom signs tell a story: for instance, that expectations of gender inclusivity may be a recent phenomenon at U-M or that people who might use that bathroom are recent arrivals, who have not been expected.[53]

Even though I immediately upon my arrival at Michigan noticed the gender-neutral bathroom signs, and that they were different in material, style, and presentation from the more permanently affixed maroon signage, my account above shows that there were many features of their materiality and presence that I elided entirely and did not move into active awareness or conscious meaning making until I had already been thinking about and moving past them on a regular basis for months. This happened despite that I had been writing about and thinking about signs of disability for years. Even as these bathroom signs call attention to certain kinds of access and presume certain kinds of bodies will be navigating this space, they also make patently clear some of the erasures and exclusions regularly enacted within this space.

How do various kinds of sensory input generated from materiality—including of bodies and texts—come to pass through perceptual apparatuses and materialize phenomena? To answer this, we can learn from work on markedness and unmarkedness in cognitive sociology,[54] which shows how orientations to social categories are shaped by collective attention, a sociological concept that excavates how people learn to build a perceptual apparatus that enables them to navigate their world. Perception is always in some ways idiosyncratic and informed by individual lived experiences, but much of what is brought to attention, noticed, and cultivated, as well as what is ignored, backgrounded, or deemed irrelevant is tied to broader cultural patterns. Eviatar Zerubavel explains, "What may seem at first glance to be a strictly personal act ultimately explainable in terms of individuals' personal tendencies . . . turns out to be actually a product of patterned default assumptions that are not unique to particular individuals."[55] Disability has a complicated relationship to collective attention. Sometimes collective attention means disability is highly marked, while at other times it is assumed to be absent or goes unnoticed. Some forms of collective attention suggest patterns of signaling that can make disability more perceptible. But those perceptions are made within contexts saturated with various intersectional *dis*-attentions that influence attentional practices, such as when institutional and structural violence erases or obscures various bodyminds, or when patterns of noticing race and gender intra-act with disability.

Asia Friedman's work on collective perception and gender identification unpacks how sensory input of others' bodies participates in perception of gender. Friedman examines the legibility and normativity of a binary gender system that shapes what many people determine to be relevant information to seek out as they negotiate social interactions. The dominance of this binary gender system in the United States, for instance, leads people to actively seek out cues that will signal information about others' gender identifications. As Friedman explains, "When we visually perceive someone as male or female, their materiality passes through one or more mental filters that sift and sort the body, marking certain details as 'relevant' and important to note, and others as 'irrelevant' and 'uninformative.' The result is a visual perception in which certain bodily details get foregrounded, while others are backgrounded and unseen or technically seen but not consciously noticed."[56]

For example, both hairstyles and the presence/absence of facial hair emerged in Friedman's interviews with blind people and with transgender people as highly relevant for identifying people as male or female, and consequently, hairstyles and facial hair were actively noticed and attended to. In turn, other kinds of readily available perceptual information, such as the shape of a person's elbow or the appearance of their shin, was rarely remarked upon or noticed. In Friedman's terms, that information is "filtered out" of awareness, revealing a process by which perceptual apparatuses are continually built and rebuilt according to what people orient to as relevant or useful. As a socially motivated process, such perceptual filtering reveals how material reality is shaped by what we are taught to notice and collectively attend to. Friedman puts it this way:

> The body does not tell us which details to look for; rather, we construct the body in the shape of our expectations by the act of looking for socially relevant features. In the case of sex, we do not simply *see*

human bodies; we *look for* "male" and "female" bodily cues. Because we expect sex differences, that is the information we seek out, and thus what "nature discloses." Of course, what unavoidably remains *unnoticed* are the evidence and details that would support other perceptions and categorizations—and by extension other social worlds, organized around different rules of relevance.[57]

Various social models—assumptions and orientations that motivate our looking and our interpretation of sensory input—lead to the emergence of particular phenomena and not others. Emergent phenomena are always shifting depending on the variety and forms of sensory input people take in as well as the cultural and collective modes of attending that influence how that input is processed. This sensory input further intra-acts with complex factors that shape how people perceive, including our own identities, lived experiences, relationships, and environments, and all of these forms of perception participate in materializing disability.

While this description of perceptual apparatuses acknowledges multiple modes of sensory perception and attentional capacities, these practices are not infinite. Zerubavel describes perception as a "zero-sum game," a point Friedman amplifies in reminding us that "seeing something *as* something means *not* seeing the other possibilities."[58] In subsequent work, she develops these attentional practices further, using the literal and figurative concept of the blind spot to illustrate numerous ways that human perceptual apparatuses fail to perceive what may be readily available for perception. The concept of the blind spot refers to a small hole in human visual fields created by scotomas where the optic nerve connects to the retina. We are generally unaware of our blind spots because our brains fill in the missing information to reveal an uninterrupted visual field. The figure of the blind spot has been widely mobilized, notably by psychologists Mahzarin R. Banaji and Anthony Greenwald, to illustrate how implicit cognitive biases help perpetuate inequality.[59] For Friedman, the figure of the blind spot helps illustrate how individual perceptions are consciously and nonconsciously shaped by cultural and collective practices of perception, thus invoking blindness to point to what is literally not seen, but also metaphorically to reference a full array of perceptual practices that materialize phenomena.[60]

I understand the resonance associated with the blind-spot metaphor in pointing to the many ways that perceptual practices attend to some details while eliding or ignoring others, just as I elided entirely the "Orientation Michigan" border and many of the details embedded in the bathroom signs described above. Yet, it presents a problem for robustly materializing disability in ways beyond visual apprehension of phenomena. Visual perception has dominated disability theorizing that explores the perceptibility of bodies.[61] This dominance is further upheld by metaphorical associations deeply embedded in our discursive and theoretical practices, a point Amy Vidali makes in her critique of Lakoff and Johnson's "seeing is knowing" metaphor[62] and reinforced by the sheer array of descriptive terms that draw from visual perception to describe scholarly or analytical work (e.g., "zoom," "focus," "develop," "pan," "illustrate," and "illuminate," among many others). Friedman notes that these practices are supported by sociological research showing that "visual information has disproportionately high truth status compared with the other senses."[63] However, like Friedman, I would like to encourage exploration of other modes of sensory perception. Despite the utility and resonance that the blind-spot metaphor might have, it can ultimately obscure resonances among forms of perception not as readily evoked, such as some of the ways that the blind people that Friedman interviewed indicated that they perceived male and female bodies drawing on touch (softness of skin, texture of clothing), scent (perfumes, food, deodorant), sound (voices, shoes on a hard floor), and more. We need to build new conceptual languages that deepen our understandings of the many forms of sensory perception that participate in disability's emergence. I will suggest some possibilities for this at the conclusion of this chapter, although I also hope and expect readers of this book will take this in all kinds of different directions, building on many creative and scholarly projects currently experimenting to build this vocabulary.

Materializing Signs of Disability

To conclude this chapter, I offer two examples of a signs-of-disability analysis that draws on the theoretical vocabulary of *dis*-attention, filtering, and perceptual apparatus that I have been forwarding thus far so as to illustrate how these concepts work together. My first example takes up physical objects and bodily figures that are frequently taken to represent or point to disability, while the second moves away from these iconic and often metonymic figures to consider shifting environmental cues and behaviors. With "signs of disability," I do not intend to suggest that orienting to disability is now or ever will be a matter of "knowing the signs," as many awareness campaigns call upon people to do. These campaigns often build on modes of noticing built through specialized knowledge (e.g., know the signs of a heart attack or of drowning or of depression) and suggest that learning to perceive in the right way(s) will materialize particular phenomena. However, as I hope the following examples will show, signs of disability are not about awareness, nor do they conceptualize knowledge or information or meaning as things or possibilities that can be spread around like butter on toast. I am thus forwarding here an always-ongoing, ever-shifting process of learning, negotiating, and attending that is less focused on specific signs to look for/at and that instead highlights dynamic folding, enfolding, and refolding practices of dominant and disabled *dis*-attentions.[64]

Signifying Objects: My Hearing Aid

My hearing aids matter. I feel them behind my ear and my ear molds often make my ear canal feel itchy. They amplify sound—quite a lot—so that I can hear conversational utterances. They recognize pitches I cannot hear at all (such as those used by many fire alarms) and move those sounds into pitches that I can hear. They are highly complex, technologically sophisticated computers manipulating how I perceive aural input through my ears, a phenomenon Steph Ceraso calls "earing."[65] These feelings and perceptions all matter for how I interact in the world.

Sometimes my hearing aids are openly discussed or negotiated in an interaction, as when I might use my hand to gesture toward my ears if I think someone has not noticed that I am deaf. In these moments, I am pointing to a difference that I perceive between how my interlocutor and I may be orienting to our interaction—I know that I am deaf, but my interlocutor might not. I am also acting on the assumption that *if* my interlocutor learns that I am deaf, they will orient differently, behave differently. But even when nobody comments on, gestures towards, or directs their gaze upon my hearing aids, my hearing aids nevertheless influence unfolding interactions. Having aural input come through my ears affects my sense of how much noise is happening in the background as well as whether someone is speaking to me even if I am not looking at them. They also matter in subtle ways: sometimes there is a lot of humidity in the air, and I can hear a crackling through my aids that interferes with the conversational sounds I am trying to discern. Sometimes my interlocutors adjust their behavior after noticing my hearing aids in ways that I do not pick up on. Sometimes my hearing aid will emit a brief high-pitched squeal when sound escapes from the ear mold, often when I am eating, chewing gum, or wearing a hat that covers part of my ears.

Because I wear my hearing aids almost every waking hour, I have built a way of moving and being in the world with them that assumes their presence, and that is disrupted when I find myself without the auditory input they provide. However, building relationships and friendships with other deaf academics, some of whom wear hearing aids, some of whom have cochlear implants, and some of whom do not wear amplification devices at all, all of us embracing, resisting, and performing different relationships to channels of sound and silence, has led me in middle age to increasingly explore the different sensory environment that emerges when I purposefully do not wear my hearing aids. In turn, I am coming to find myself enjoying not wearing them and I am building new relations not only with people who are coming into my life but also with objects like my hearing aids. The possibilities go on and on, and they are influenced by a dynamic and ever-changing set of potentials.

Despite the regularity with which objects pointing to disability are represented as decontextualized icons, my hearing aids are almost never perceived apart from my body.[66] And even if I am not wearing them, they are always perceived in *some* context, some material arrangement that makes them available for perception. Their materiality is entangled with processes of observation and boundary enactment that lead them to appear in particular ways, or even, not-appear. That I am white, that my hearing aids are extremely expensive, that I both identify and am generally identified by others as female all matter to how my hearing aids appear and take shape. These factors of my appearance and bodily materiality intra-act with my hearing aids to make them differently perceptible or imperceptible in different contexts and relations. Some deaf academics I know have brightly colored ear molds, while mine are something of a translucent color. Even though my hair is short, I have chosen hearing aids that are similar in color to my hair and blend in, rather than contrast. What others immediately orient to about my body and my appearance in shared social (and virtual) spaces is shaped by intra-actions within those environments that ultimately materialize and enact boundaries around phenomena while leaving aside other possible materializations.

Thinking about my hearing aid doing interactional work as a sign of disability involves noticing not just the hearing aid but also how it functions as part of my material embodiment in conjunction with other aspects of my physical presence that an interlocutor might perceive. A hearing aid is not in and of itself a sign of disability. Not everyone who wears a hearing aid identifies as disabled; not all hearing aids material- ize disability.[67] So part of the line of questioning here involves, *When and how does my hearing aid function as a sign of disability? Put another way, when and how does disability materialize in relation to the hear- ing aid?* Materializing disability involves the intra-action of a perceptual (measuring) apparatus and perceived sensory input that is interpreted and accorded meaning. What sensory aspects of my presence do others around me perceive? What auditory, visual, tactile, olfactory, and taste inputs do people take in and interpret to materialize disability? What perceptual apparatuses do they employ in paying attention, and how do forms of *dis*-attention and collective attention shape these orientations? How does my hearing aid agentially intra-act in these contexts? How does it shape my own behaviors and practices?

I have spent most of my academic career in working environments where I am the only person who openly identifies as deaf. But in recent years this orientation has shifted as I have spent more time engaging with deaf colleagues and seeking out increased opportunities to be around other deaf academics. It also shifted when a disability studies colleague whose work engages significantly with deafness and rhetoric as well as another deaf colleague were hired at my institution. I spent thirteen years at the University of Delaware—a period of relative professional stability that enabled me to perceive what happens differently when I am new (as I was at Michigan during my scholar-in-residence period) than when I have built long-standing relationships with colleagues who have some familiarity with my presence and modes of participation. These are dynamic ecologies. I cannot point to my hearing aids and say "this is what they mean" because how they are perceived, what is perceived, and how that sensory input intra-acts with a perceptual apparatus all materialize differently. Different kinds of hearing aids differently signal. How and what they signal depends on the everyday and specialized knowledges and forms of being that shape perceptual apparatuses.

Now, lest I seem to be suggesting that signs of disability inhere on persons and/or material artifacts, let me share a second example that helps illustrate the dynamic ecologies in which signs of disability function. This one involves my ongoing relationships with what Sean Zdenek has called "reading sounds" in his groundbreaking book on the rhetorics of closed-captioning.[68]

Environmental Disability: The Captioning Logo

Since its early development, closed-captioning was often indicated with a logo printed next to TV or movie listings in the newspaper or on the side of VHS tapes or DVDs that looked like a small rectangle with a tail hanging from it. For a long stretch of my life—until I was in my midtwenties, in fact—I was highly attuned to this symbol as an indicator of whether I would be able to watch a TV program or movie. When I was a child, my family had a closed-caption decoder that was about the size of a large VCR. This metal and faux-wood box with UHF and VHF dials on it connected to our TV set and when turned on, enabled the display of captions at the bottom of my TV screen for TV shows and movies that had embedded closed-captioning. The squarish icon indicated whether a show had closed captions or not. In the early days of closed-captioning, only a few shows were captioned. I remember scouring TV listings looking for this square conversation bubble and was vigilant about checking for it whenever I would borrow a video from the library or the video store, and in this process, I became an expert on where these icons would likely be found, often on the back or the side of the cassette sleeve.

Now, this little square with a tail does not by itself index disability. But it was a sign, to me and to many others, that could point to an orientation to disability. It indexed whether I would likely be able to watch this video or show, although whether I would be able to watch it depended also on the presence of a closed-caption decoder box; on weather conditions that sometimes affected TV signals and interfered with closed-caption display; on social environments and others' feelings and behaviors around captions. For instance, my older brother regularly turned off the caption decoder anytime he thought I was not looking (all this involved was pressing a single button on the decoder box), and for a long, long time it was common for people around me to protest that captions on their screen ruined their experience of watching TV, leaving me to feel torn between demanding my own access to the social activity of TV watching and the desire not to take away from others' enjoyment.

Over time, I became familiar with which video distributors and which network channels were most likely to consistently caption their programming. I also began to be able to make predictions about captioning availability without having to seek out a definitive sign specifically indicating that something I wanted to watch was captioned. Then, in 1990, the US Congress passed the Television Decoder Circuitry Act, which mandated that all new television sets thirteen inches or larger sold in the United States contain caption-decoding technology.[69] This law had dramatic material consequences for the ways that I socialized and interacted with people, activities that often involved having a TV on even if watching a sporting event, TV show, or movie was not the central activity. I no longer needed to have the bulky decoder box, and I was not limited to consuming captioned content only at my own house, at my friend Vanessa's house,[70] or at the homes of other friends who were also deaf.

As captioning has become more common, as multiple audiences have come to recognize the benefits captioning brings to their experience of watching TV, and as video technologies have changed, my relationship to this logo has shifted: I no longer look for that caption icon but rather for subtitles. I also look for the way subtitles are labeled: if it just says "English" rather than "English SDH" (subtitled for the deaf and hard of hearing), I worry about the kind of access I will get to what Zdenek calls "rhetorically significant sounds," such as the ringing of a phone or ominous background noises that might orient watchers to action happening within a scene. One way disability materializes—or rather, dominant *dis*-attention materializes—is when I am watching a movie where deaf people are not the primary audience for the captions. In *Schindler's List*, for instance, almost the entire movie is in German, with English subtitles throughout. But when the American soldiers come to the camp at the end of the movie, there are no captions for the English words they speak. The different means for captioning music, from a single musical note to parentheticals describing the music to a caption naming the artist and the song to transcription of the lyrics, all reveal different ways that caption readers are imagined as audiences, only some of which overlap with disability.[71] I have lost count of the number of movies I have watched where anything that is sung is ignored entirely by the captions. And whether rhetorically significant sounds appear in the captions depends on whether the captioning audience is imagined as deaf, or as just needing access to the English words that are spoken.

The logos have shifted, the technologies are dramatically different, and people's familiarity with closed captioning has come to a point where I can now reasonably assume that something I want to watch will be captioned, and I rarely find myself looking for a caption icon or logo for programming offered through TV and film networks. However, while my attention to captioning logos has waned, the rise of Internet video, live streaming, and the sheer proliferation of user-created content on YouTube, TikTok, Vimeo, and other video-sharing websites has led me to seek different cues and signals to ascertain accessibility in those spaces. As I write this book, these technologies have advanced to the point that now, rather than ignoring Internet videos entirely, I seek out cues such as whether the video is a single speaker using microphones and other effective sound production tools, whether the video is hosted on a site with automatic captioning resources, whether a TV station or network is doing the streaming, and more. As a deaf person, I am always looking for signs of disability—the materialization of disability as something to which video creators and distributors are attending.

This example illustrates how signs of disability can differently materialize within different contexts. It further suggests that what constitutes disability is not simply a matter of moving concepts, focal objects, or definitions from one context to another and applying them or studying their mattering in different contexts. Rather, it involves reconstituting the category anew within different intra-actions. It involves understanding how beings are and might be oriented, how perceptual apparatuses condition forms of noticing and of not-noticing, and how new ways of attending to disability can emerge. My movements and orientations to the caption logo resonate with what rhetorical theorist Marilyn Cooper has described as neurophenomenological feedback loops in which beings move through the world gathering information that then influences subsequent actions and movements.[72] (More on this in chapter 2.) This continual process of sorting and organizing information according to the perception and interpretation of sensory input, including others' material and embodied presence, is precisely the means of building a perceptual apparatus for disability. Within such feedback loops, beings learn what information is relevant to help them interpret and organize the world more efficiently, and they treat some kinds of input as relevant while eliding other information streams as irrelevant or unimportant.

Learning from Signs of Disability

The two examples presented above show how a signs-of-disability analysis might proceed, storying not about figures identified as disabled but about how and what we perceive at different times and in different relations. I conclude here by asking two questions: How can we learn from our orientation to signs of disability? And how might signs of disability be incorporated into everyday practices of noticing, to resist dominant dis-attentions? To respond, I again turn to Friedman's work on perception and filtering, which I will describe in terms of absences, erasures, and elisions emerging from both dominant and disabled dis-attentions. What we do not perceive can be associated with two general perceptual strategies: habituation and focusing, which each describe various practices of backgrounding and foregrounding various kinds of sensory input.

In habituation, many details may be taken for granted and assumed, rather than actively noticed. Habituation is in many ways connected to cognitive efficiency. Given how many details there are for noticing and the limits of our attentional apparatuses, we often benefit from being able to background many of our perceptions,[73] and Friedman suggests that habituation might more usefully be described in terms of a field rather than a "spot." In contrast to habituation's practices of backgrounding, in which "tacit social value is associated with what is unattended, rather than what is noticed,"[74] focusing instead suggests a lack of attention "to socially irrelevant complexity, ambiguity, and anomaly, rather than the normative and taken-for-granted."[75] To learn to perceive what we may not be perceiving, Friedman suggests that one strategy is to consider ourselves strangers in an environment and notice things anew, much as I did when, on the brink of leaving Michigan, I took another look at the gender-inclusive bathroom signs I had been passing all year. Such strategies may be particularly important for calling attention to different practices of perception at work within collective scenes. For instance, feelings of comfort and discomfort are often motivated by perceptual practices not always explicitly identified or named. Exploring these feelings and where they may be rooted or connected may be a strategy for bringing backgrounded structures into more conscious awareness.[76]

Focusing takes a different approach to cognitive efficiency than habituation. We learn from others around us what details are relevant for categorizing and grouping things together, leading us to focus on and seek out those details while *dis*-attending others. In terms of disability, then, we are often invited to notice disability in special education, in various accoutrements such as wheelchairs, hearing aids, and white canes, and with particular kinds of bodies. But we are not as well poised to readily recognize the complex dynamics in which race and disability mutually constitute one another, or which treat some phenomena as common and perhaps unimportant in some bodies while remarking on their surprisingness or importance in other bodies. By "lumping" groups together, or by "splitting" them in particular ways on the basis of assumptions about relevant details, we can reinforce stereotypes and dominant orientations to particular categories. In *Hidden in Plain Sight*, Zerubavel suggests that we might "unlump" or "unsplit" these categories in order to understand the boundaries and relationships underlying their (lack of) coherence.[77] The conceptual work involved in these efforts, Friedman notes, "is a constant dynamic process of filtering out the ambiguous and irrelevant, involving subtle adjustments of attention to keep the necessary [*dis*-attentions] in place."[78] Perhaps one of the most important strategies I will encourage in this book involves engaging with disabled forms of *dis*-attention, particularly forms of sensory perception that may, for many of us, be backgrounded or elided given the dominance of the visual. Again, here I learn from Friedman, who notes that a key argument emerging from her interviews with blind people "is that dominant everyday conceptions of sex are based mostly on visual data and therefore exclude all the information available through the other senses, much of which conveys a great deal of ambiguity."[79]

Grappling with the ambiguity often reflected in signs of disability and their mutability is a site of both great potential and challenge. Learning to perceive disability is not an act of altruism or a means of simply noticing forms of access and accessibility in your surround: it is part of building a world that assumes disability's presence and participation and is poised to grapple with the tensions and questions that consequently emerge. The rest of this book will attempt to nudge us in these directions, beginning by taking up in the next chapter how signs of disability disclose within contexts suffused with dominant *dis*-attentions.

2

Disclosing

As we encounter signs of disability all around us, how do we learn to understand them? Another way to ask that question might be, What stories do these signs tell about disability? How do these stories, produced by material bodies and circulated as material artifacts, matter to and shape disability's ongoing dynamism in the world? A materialist theory of disclosure can help us respond to these questions. In *The Material of Knowledge*, Susan Hekman forwards such a theory, explaining that "disclosure entails that perspectives/concepts/theories matter—that they are our means of accessing reality. But," she adds, "disclosure also entails that we do not constitute that reality with our concepts, but rather portray it in varying ways. An important aspect of this understanding is that the reality, like the object in the photograph or the subject of the scientist's experiment, is agentic. It pushes back, it effects the result."[1]

Hekman's account of disclosure stresses not just the mattering of how people name, describe, create, and recreate phenomena through the stories we tell but also the work that "the object in the photograph or the subject of the scientist's experiment" does in "push[ing] back, effect[ing] the result." This understanding of material agency, in turn, suggests our responsibility to learn to *dis*-attend in ways that comport with the world's disclosures, to resist dominant forms of *dis*-attention while inviting disabled *dis*-attentions.

The tension between what is disclosed within an environment and what is made available for perception is powerfully illustrated in a pair of photographs taken and shared with me by Tara Wood. The first shows a large, carefully trimmed bush planted in front of a red brick building on the University of Oklahoma campus.

The photograph's framing is a bit odd as the bush dominates the photograph, taking up more than half the image. This photo reveals dominant *dis*-attentions that elide disability because there is a wheelchair logo/inaccessible entrance sign in this photograph. It is not easy to

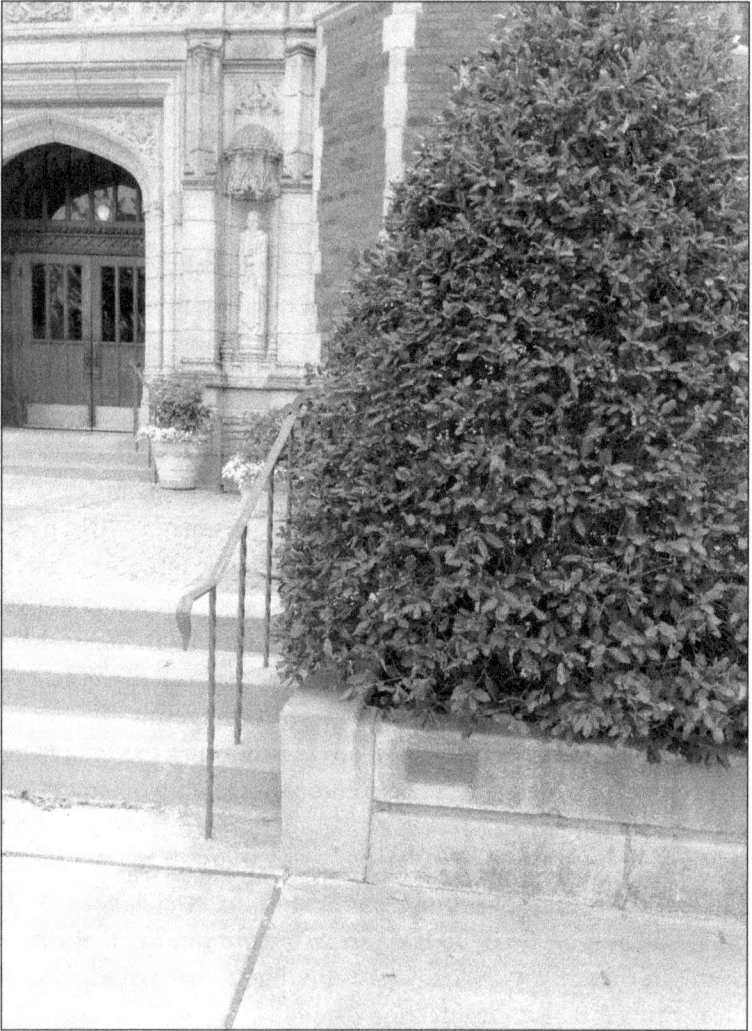

Figure 2.1. Bush and Red Brick Building. Image description: A large, carefully trimmed bush planted in front of a red brick building on the University of Oklahoma campus. The building's heavy-looking double wooden doors are framed by ornate stone. Immediately to the left of the bush are three stone steps leading to a landing and then more steps in front of the doors. Norman, Oklahoma. (Photo by Tara Wood.)

perceive, and if you missed it, you are not alone. Figure 2.2 shows an enlarged section of a second, close-up photo Wood took of the bush. Only when I focus intensely on this enlarged photo can I make out portions of a blue background and some white and red lines among the bush's leaves and branches. What I can see indicates that this is a blue sign featuring the International Symbol of Access, a stick figure in a wheelchair, with a red circle and a slash through it. Finding this sign buried within the

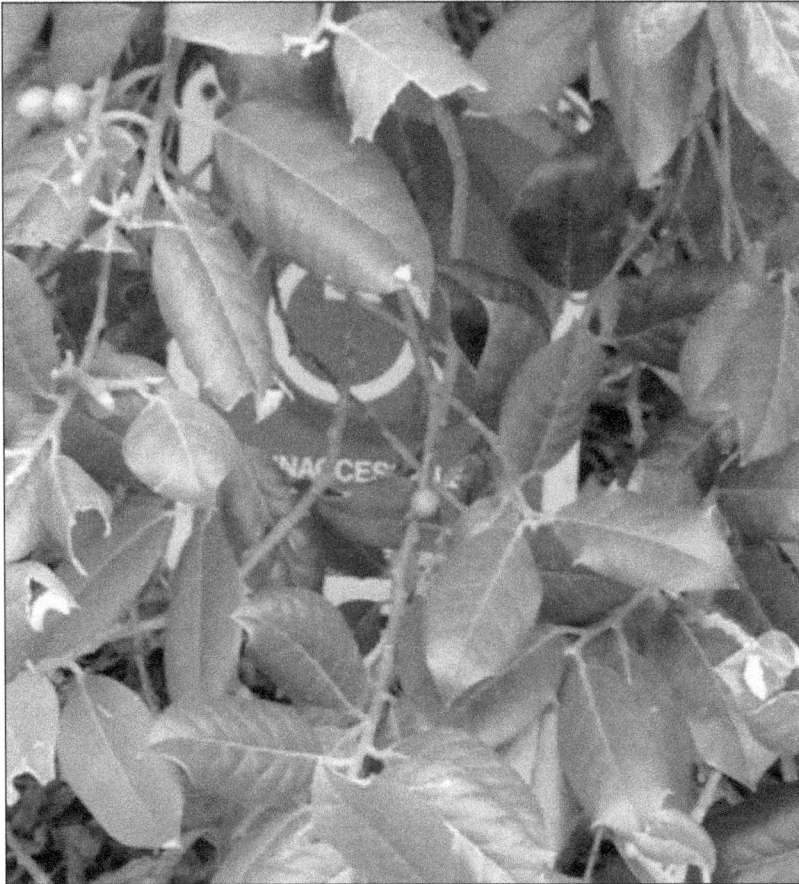

Figure 2.2. Enlargement of Close-Up Photo of Bush in Figure 2.1 Image description: Within a bush's branches and leaves, portions of a blue background and some white lines peek out. Parts of a red circle and slash surround fragments of the wheelchair icon and white letters reading "NA CES LE" peer between branches and leaves. Norman, Oklahoma. (Photo by Tara Wood.)

bush is all the more surprising because it has been carefully gardened and trimmed into a conical shape: this is no jungle-like overgrowth that often obscures road signs. In an essay about dilemmas of inclusive architecture, Margaret Price looks at a very similar sign, likewise obscured in shrubbery, to ask questions about whom access and inclusion are truly intended for.[2] These questions are relevant to ask about this sign as well: it would be nearly impossible for anyone to casually pass the bush and apprehend a sign in its midst—except, perhaps, someone who needs the information provided by the sign and who might be scouring their environment for cues regarding an accessible entrance.

Dis-attention emerges as the scene might appear as just an ordinary scene. Signs of disability are not expected, and they are not noticed, and this not-noticing is, as Tanya Titchkosky explains, unsurprising, commonplace, quotidian.[3] *Dis*-attention also emerges through the carefully trimmed bush. There are many possible stories here: maybe another sign made the one in the bush redundant and rather than being removed, the sign was left in the bush, perhaps even forgotten. Maybe the bush grew too large, and in its unruliness obscured the sign, thus consigning it to near-oblivion. *Dis*-attention also emerges in the vantage point of the photographer, whose awkward framing in the first image offers a clue that there is maybe something about the bush leading it to get near-center stage. We need to perceive the steps and the lead-up to the heavy wooden doors, as well as the fullness of the bush, to feel that there is something off here. *Dis*-attention emerges as Wood helps us peer in between the branches. Her perception of the sign was likely motivated by her own disabled practices of *dis*-attention, built through lived experiences as a disability studies scholar and as a person with intimate relationships to disability. The attentional practices she has cultivated in her life and her work help her to materialize the sign within the bush's leaves and branches.

Disability is there and yet—it is not there. Even when the sign's fragments pass through a perceptual apparatus, it will never be the only means of signaling disability in this scene: the stairs, the door, the bush, the photograph, and the accounts of the photograph all potentially enable the emergence of disability as part of an always-changing range of potential intra-actions between apparatus and reality. These signs disclose *dis*-attentions that elide disability as well as *dis*-attentions that are motivated by lived experiences of disability, and all of these stories contribute to an understanding of reality that takes shape through encounters with these photographs.

To navigate the entangled *dis*-attentions detailed here, to understand how different *dis*-attentions intra-act and shape perception and emergent phenomena, is to negotiate story. Here is another story about accessible entrance signs that shows the intra-acting effects of dominant and disabled *dis*-attentions. In this story, Tobin Siebers shares a memory of navigating to a new campus building that he had not previously visited:

> From my car, I try to scout out the location of the handicapped entrance. I spot a little blue sign with a wheelchair on it. I circle the block for twenty minutes, passing many other parking spaces while waiting for a parking place to open up near that little blue sign. I park and walk over to the door. But under that wheelchair is a tiny arrow, pointing to the left. No other writing. It seems that this is a sign telling me that this is not the handicapped entrance. The real handicapped entrance is somewhere to the left of me.[4]

In this story Siebers narrates actively seeking cues pointing to disability (just as I did with the caption logo in chapter 1), looking for information in his everyday environment that would help him determine the best means of accessing a building. But this story also highlights that implementation of such signage sometimes conveys more about dominant forms of *dis*-attention that ignore or elide disability than about *dis*-attentions that are shaped by disabled people's lived experiences. In yet another example, Amy Vidali performs a close reading of a photograph taken at the University of Nevada–Reno.[5] The photo features a blue sign with a wheelchair icon inside a red circle and with a red slash across it—the same image that appears to be on the sign in figure 2.2. The sign's positioning points to a route that is inaccessible not because of steps or impassable terrain but because the path's steep grade and street at its end make it dangerous for someone in a wheelchair to navigate. The irony in Vidali's photograph, however, is that the vantage point of the image is such that as one looks toward the horizon, the inaccessible sign seems to be positioned against UNR flags in the distance, conveying a message of the inaccessibility of not just one path but the entire campus.

In this way, disabled and dominant *dis*-attentions entangle in surprising associations that emerge as signs are placed within particular material environments and are encountered by agents practiced with different forms of *dis*-attention. A second entanglement is reflected in Siebers's assumption, as he waited for a desirable parking spot near a familiar-looking blue sign with the wheelchair logo on it, that the sign pointed toward accessibility rather than inaccessibility.

Signs that point to accessibility and inaccessibility comprise a large portion of the archive of signs of disability in public places that I have been photographing and collecting for more than six years now. Some of my interest in these signs was spurred by a 2015 visit to the University of Illinois at Urbana-Champaign, during which I was given a hotel room in the center of campus and an itinerary that included several free hours that I used to wander around. As I navigated campus, I found myself moving slowly and taking pictures at almost every turn. There were so many signs! I was especially struck by how large and visible the accessible entrance signage was. Why was this surprising to me? Because of the contrast it offered with the signage I was used to on my own campus. Figures 2.3 and 2.4 illustrate some of the differences in prominence and style in signage at UIUC and at the University of Delaware.

What underlying beliefs about signage and about disability are disclosed in the juxtaposition of these images? In asking why the buildings at UIUC have such large signage pointing to accessible entrances, we might note that many of UIUC's buildings—like the University of Michigan's Angell Hall, discussed in chapter 1—are large and imposing structures fronted with steep steps leading to their entrances.[6] Navigating to an accessible entrance can, in some cases, mean traversing several blocks to circle the building. Easily perceptible signage is, as the accounts shared by Vidali, Siebers, and Price all emphasize, important for helping people identify efficient routes to accessible entrances and pathways. But the UIUC signs' ready perceptibility is of course not the whole story. Some of the signs I was encountering seemed quite fancy: nice, large, gold signs with black lettering that were generally perceptible in approaching the building. I was impressed as I wandered around the campus, and honestly, have not been this struck by a campus's disability signage since. The UIUC signs did not seem like half-assed retrofits[7] or afterthoughts. They suggested to me that this kind of physical

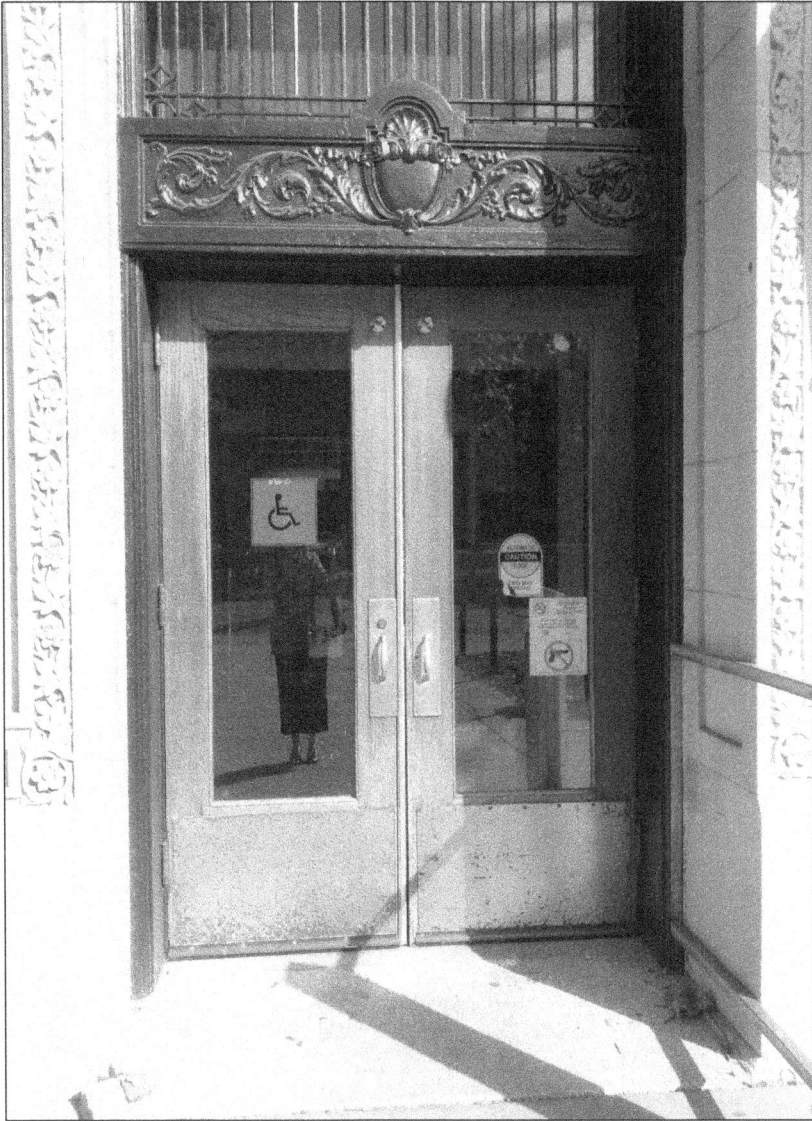

Figure 2.3. Materials Science and Engineering Building, University of Illinois, circa 2015. Image description: A building at the University of Illinois showing an ornate entrance with large double doors framed with wood and with clear glass panels in their center. A gold square with a black wheelchair logo is prominently centered on the left door while the right door features an automatic-door-opener logo and a sign indicating that guns are not allowed in campus buildings. Urbana, Illinois. (Photo by author.)

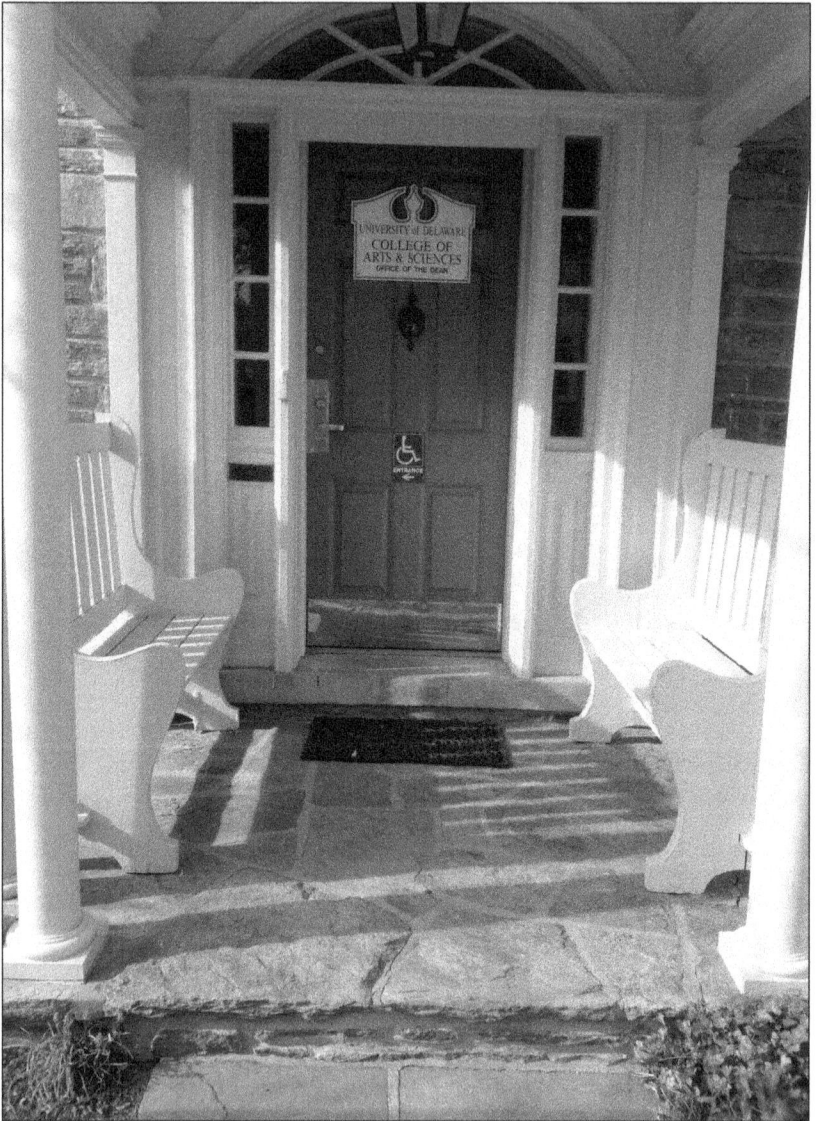

Figure 2.4. The College of Arts and Sciences, University of Delaware, circa 2013. Image description: The entrance to the College of Arts and Sciences at the University of Delaware, which shows a step onto a stone porch and another step up to the door. The door features a sign with the name of the building, and below it, to the right of the door handle, a small sign with a wheelchair icon and some text that is not clearly readable from the position of the photographer, but when one gets close enough, is revealed to be the word "Entrance" with a small arrow pointing to the left indicating an accessible entrance around the back. Newark, Delaware. (Photo by author.)

accessibility might perhaps be part of the UIUC culture, something that one generally encountered in moving through campus rather than being a "special" consideration awkwardly appended onto buildings.

When I talked about the signage with some of the UIUC faculty during my visit, one mentioned the prominence of Illinois's wheelchair basketball team. I later learned that in 1948, Illinois was the first college in the United States to establish a wheelchair basketball team[8] and that it currently boasts one of the top adaptive sports programs in the United States.[9] Having an established history of wheelchair athletics as well as a robust community of disabled athletes needing physical access to campus buildings could have been a powerful impetus for the development and placement of Illinois's signage, which was put in place before blue signs with white icons and lettering, as shown in figure 2.4, became something of a US standard. But this is just one set of possible stories— were I to have spent more than two days on the UIUC campus and were I to have a different kind of familiarity with the campus, I would have a different, potentially more nuanced story to tell about this accessible entrance signage. One early reader of this chapter, for instance, asked a number of questions about the images shared here, the answers to which would shape the stories that get told about Illinois's accessibility signage. What other stories might we tell? What else are these signs disclosing? These questions reveal that those who perceive these signs—and perhaps especially those, like me, who search for them—are always working with only partial information, telling one story, or perhaps imagining multiple stories, that are all taking shape amid their concatenation of experiences and practices of dominant and disabled *dis*-attentions.

Now I want to take some time to probe more deeply the disclosures that signs in public places, often comprised of metal, paper, plastic, or wood, make of disability. The wheelchair logo/International Symbol of Access (ISA) is by far the most prominent index of disability that I have photographed or had shared with me. It has also received the greatest attention from scholars studying disability signage. In her book *Designing Disability*, Elizabeth Guffey performs an extended historical analysis of the ISA,[10] and numerous others have unpacked various functions performed by this icon,[11] including how it conveys messages about mobility,[12] affective valences for disability,[13] and attitudes towards access.[14] The ISA is not the only public sign of disability to receive significant attention:

Alison Kafer and Eli Clare have each turned to motivational billboards to uncover problematic subtexts about disability and ableness, and Najma al Zidjaly shows how the use of a universal access symbol effectively erases representations of individual disabled people in Oman.[15] These analyses underscore the variety and range of meaning making that coalesce around the materiality of various signs. However, even as the ISA (as well as various updated configurations, such as the wheelchair logo refigured by the Accessible Icon Project)[16] has been the most prevalent sign of disability that I have collected over the last seven years, it was a different sign that first caught my attention and ultimately came to preoccupy my thinking: a yellow diamond-shaped sign that appeared in my neighborhood with the words "Deaf Person in Area" on it (figure 2.5).

For several years, I passed this sign every day (and its identical twin, down the street and facing the other direction) driving to and from work. It just appeared—I don't know when. It is very possible I passed it without even noticing it, until I did notice it. When this sign appeared, I found myself a bit *dis*-oriented. I wondered, "When did that get here?" "How long have I not noticed this?" "Will I ever know who the Deaf Person in Area is?" I laughed to myself: "Good thing I live in the neighborhood, so there actually *is* a Deaf Person in Area!" I pointed the sign out to my partner. We laughed together. I took pictures of the sign. I wrote a conference presentation about disability disclosure. In that talk,[17] I offered the sign as a metaphor for how most people think disability disclosure works: you announce, loudly, "Deaf Person in Area!" and, well, that's about it.[18] Only nobody knows what to do when they are told "Deaf Person in Area." Do they drive faster? Slower? Honk their horn? Avoid honking? Or nothing at all?

Over the last few years, this sign has worked on and through me in numerous ways: I have talked about this sign in a lot of places with a lot of people. I have taken pictures of more yellow diamond-shaped signs. I have asked others to share pictures of signs. More than a year after the original "Deaf Person in Area" sign entered my conscious awareness, I encountered two additional signs: one off a side street near the first one and a second planted directly in front of a neatly trimmed suburban house in a small and low-trafficked cul-de-sac (figures 2.6 and 2.7). I used a cropped version of figure 2.5 as the background for my computer's desktop (figure 2.8), as the cover image for a Facebook group, and as

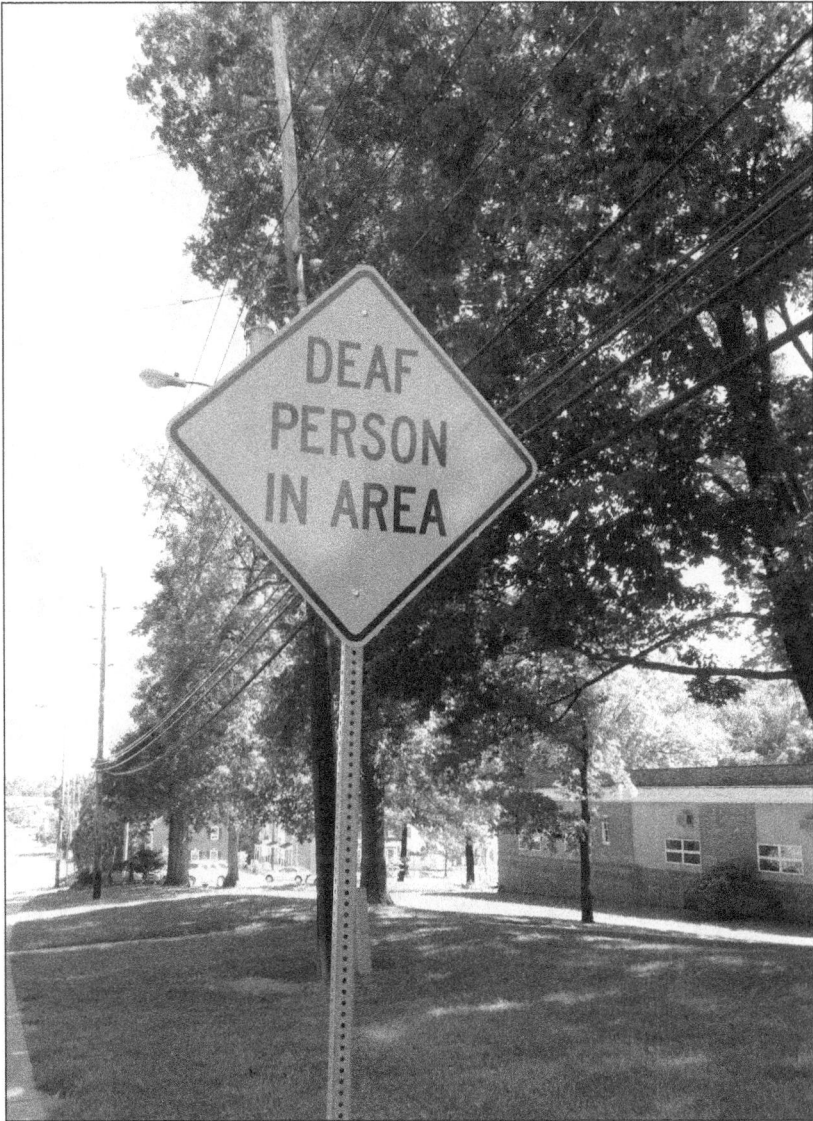

Figure 2.5. "Deaf Person in Area" Sign on Main Road. Image description: A yellow diamond-shaped road sign that reads "Deaf Person in Area" along a well-trafficked road. In the background are large trees with many leaves on them, telephone poles and wires, and a squat brick community center. Newark, Delaware. (Photo by author.)

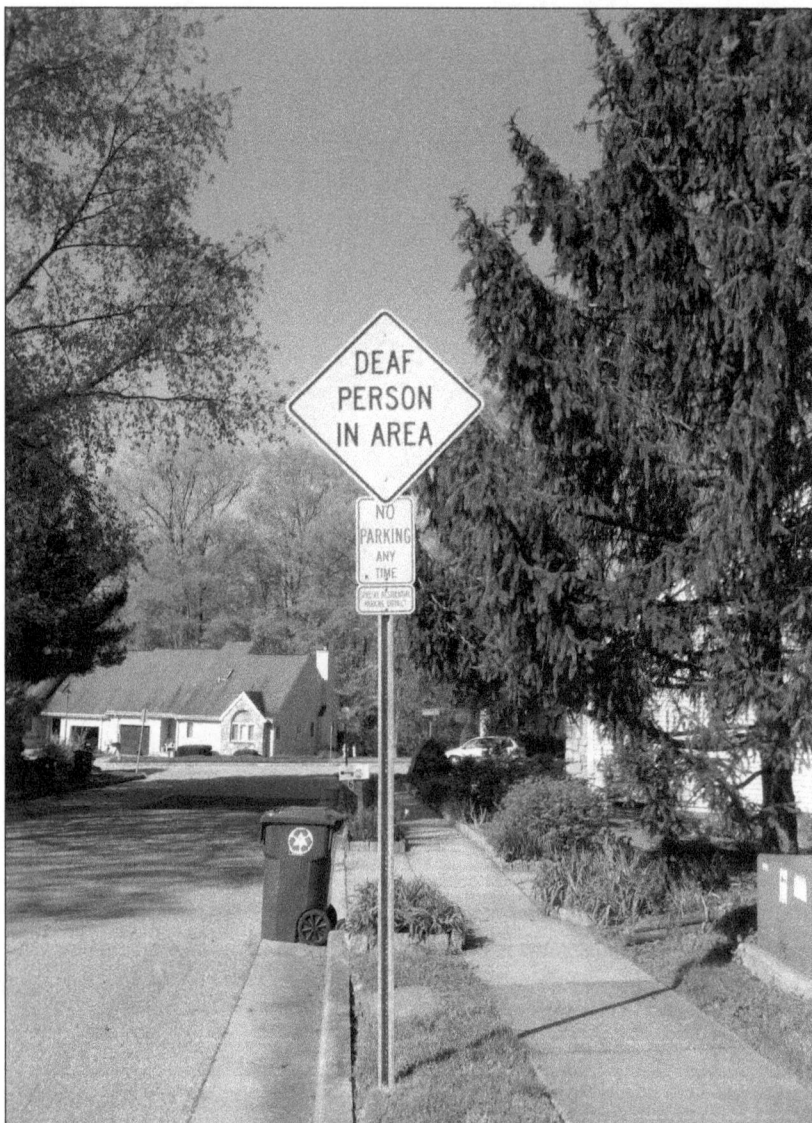

Figure 2.6. "Deaf Person in Area Sign" off Main Road. Image description: A yellow diamond-shaped sign reading "Deaf Person in Area" planted on the grassy median between sidewalk and street on a relatively quiet suburban street. Just below it is a "No Parking Any Time" sign and a smaller sign saying, "Special Residential Parking District." A large pine tree takes up much of the right side of the image, and a single-family home is in the distance. Newark, Delaware. (Photo by author.)

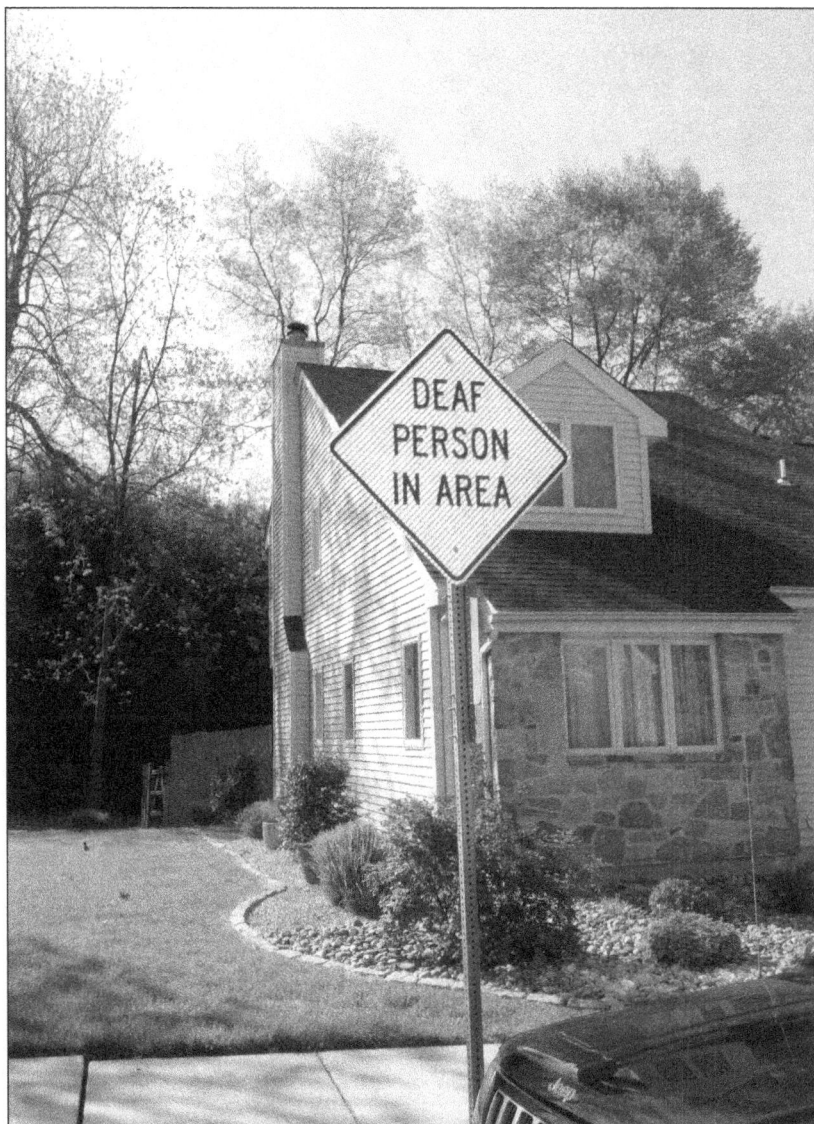

Figure 2.7. "Deaf Person in Area" Sign in Front of House. Image description: A yellow diamond-shaped sign reading "Deaf Person in Area" planted on the grassy median between sidewalk and street directly in front of a well-manicured single-family Cape Cod–style home. Does the Deaf Person in Area live here? Newark, Delaware. (Photo by author.)

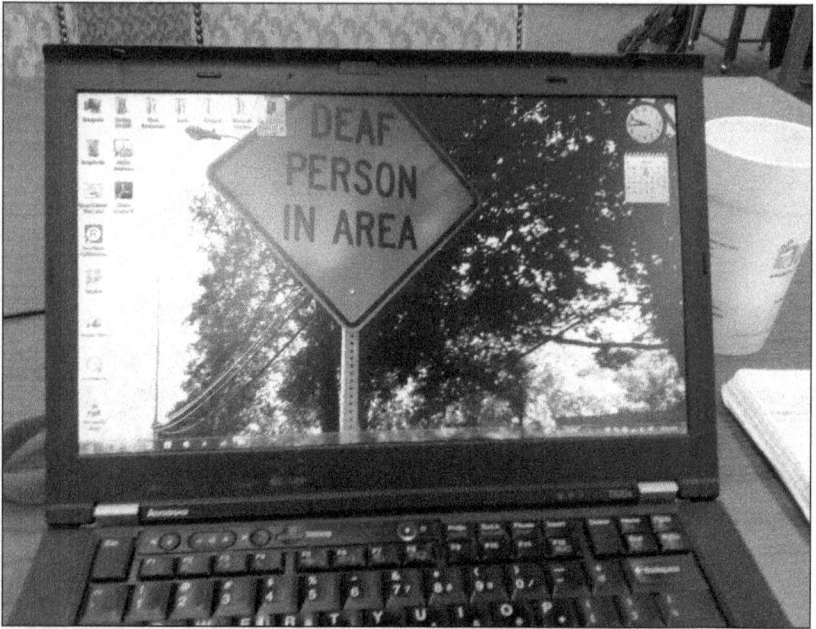

Figure 2.8. "Deaf Person in Area" Sign as Laptop Background. Image description: My laptop on a table in my university's library, showing a closely cropped image of the "Deaf Person in Area" sign being used as my laptop's background. A Styrofoam coffee cup and the corner of a notebook are on the right side of the image. Newark, Delaware. (Photo by author.)

a recurring image on my academic website. Not only was I driving past the original "Deaf Person in Area" sign on a daily basis, but its images were circulating in numerous spheres of my life. The sign influenced me and shaped my perception. I thought about what it might mean to have a sign announcing "Deaf Person in Area" and when such signs might be needed and what other kinds of signs might be at work in my conscious and nonconscious perceptions. As the "Deaf Person in Area" sign circulated in my world, I began to think, "Should I have a sign? Where would I put it?" It did not take long before I started thinking of myself as a living embodiment of a "Deaf Person in Area" sign. My very presence and participation—everywhere and everywhen—involve myriad intra-acting and ongoing disclosures of deafness, and the signs do not always take shape the way others around me might expect.

While the yellow diamond-shaped sign is no longer in my neighborhood, it has not left me since our first encounter. Meditating on the phrase "Deaf Person in Area" led me to wonder how disability materializes as I negotiate everyday interactions at work, at home, with friends, with family, with strangers, with colleagues, with acquaintances, on the phone, on email, in person, on video conferences. Initially, I latched on to largely visually identifiable means by which disability or deafness might become apparent: my hearing aids; hands moving in sign language; captioning displayed on a TV screen; spoken or signed utterances such as "I'm deaf" or pointing to my ears. But the list quickly got more and more complicated. Perceiving my deafness could involve various kinds of auditory input such as the quality and tone of my voice alongside listeners' experiences with or knowledge of various kinds of accents. People might also notice pauses or the pacing of an interaction or recognize the use of particular terms or phrases. Indeed, the range of things others could perceive, using all kinds of sensory practices, quickly became limitless. And all of this perception is further shaped by both dominant and disabled dis-attentions that cue particular kinds of noticing. Disability perceptibility thus depends on numerous factors, including the environmental surround and ecological context, agents' short- and long-term interactional goals, and their emerging and ongoing relationships with other beings and their surround (see also chapter 1).[19]

Here I suggest disability as an emergent phenomenon that is disclosed through intra-actions between human perceptual apparatuses and the world's materiality converted into sensory input. Disability disclosures in turn shape emerging and dynamic cultural orientations to disability. In turning to disclosures made by material artifacts such as accessible entrance and yellow diamond-shaped "Deaf Person in Area" signs, my hope is to reveal the pervasiveness of dominant forces of dis-attention as well as their entanglement with dis-attentions motivated by disabled epistemologies. To do this, I first link Hekman's material concept of disclosure with Rebecca Sanchez's notion of "doing disability with others"[20] and use this formulation to show the yellow diamond-shaped signs disclosing relationships among disability, race, and animality. I conclude by gesturing toward the ethical responsibilities that our dis-attentions call to awareness.

Material Disclosures

I noted at the start of this chapter that when I first encountered the "Deaf Person in Area" sign, it revealed itself to me as funny. Other deaf people have reported similar reactions: in a blog post about a "Deaf Pedestrians" sign complete with flashing lights near Gallaudet University, Tonya Stremlau wrote, "When I drive by, I do sometimes irrationally feel like I should get out and walk by the sign, just to give it a raison d'etre."[21] Similarly, in "How Not to Be a Dick to a Deaf Person," Kelly Dougher captioned a photo of a "Deaf Child in Area" sign with, "This sign is still on my street even though I turned 18 ages ago. This is the first time it has made itself useful."[22] But as I engaged more widely with the sign, it disclosed to me in quite different ways. Most people I talked to did not experience the sign as funny or ridiculous. These were occasionally difficult conversations. Sometimes I would feel a bit indignant: "Really? Do you think I should have a 'Deaf Person in Area' sign in front of my house? Should I have one at the door to my office? Should I carry one everywhere I go so that everyone always knows that there's a Deaf Person in Area?" "No, no, no," people would respond. "*You* don't need a sign, but there are lots of *other* deaf people who do. You're not like them. You're different." Here I have to pause to refuse the exceptionalism implied by these comments. In the ongoing dynamics of intra-activity, there are no clear, once-and-for-all distinctions that can be drawn between me and other deaf people.

I carry with me many "Deaf Person in Area" signs, and can even be understood as a living, breathing, moving "Deaf Person in Area" sign. Many features of my physical presence and of my behavior within social spaces can be signs of disability. And yet, there is a great deal of ambiguity behind any potential sign of disability. None has a direct line to meaning or representation. Understanding these perceptions as "disclosures" in the word's conventional meaning ignores what Sanchez calls the "crucial difference between sharing information about one's body and being interpolated into a particular identity based on the (mis)perceptions of others."[23] Instead, Sanchez's articulation of doing disability with others puts the onus on an ongoing process that might be launched by multisensory perceptions of material artifacts and bodies but that is not its culmination. While such processes may seem to begin with the perception of materiality in myriad ways, there is no "beginning" or "conclusion." There are just ongoing iterative processes of intra-actions that emerge phenomena and disclose properties or boundaries.

Disclosures, like stories, are significant in their iterations. Repeated encounters have left marks on me and have been consequential for my movements in the world. In other writing, I have tried to understand the significance of such encounters. In "On Rhetorical Agency," I wrote about the experience of having colleagues at different times, with different degrees of familiarity with me, in different environments ask me to account for my deafness in my scholarly writing. In *Toward a New Rhetoric of Difference*, I turned to recurrent encounters in which different aspects of my identity—wearing glasses, being deaf, being white, and being female—each materialize as significant at different times and in different ways and in different encounters and in different environments. Each of these stories has come to me through singular encounters within sociomaterial environments and the dynamic movement of everyday life. They have thickened and thinned, taken on different resonances, and morphed and shaped as the multispecies beings and object beings around me and I mutually change.

Understanding myself as a "Deaf Person in Area" sign opens up numerous resonances and questions. How does the body function as a sign, making disability available for others' perception? How does deafness, often described as a nonapparent or invisible disability, become perceptible within everyday interactional scenes? How do various kinds of material artifacts, running the full gamut from hearing aids to buttons and pins to various kinds of medicines to mobility aids to nearly anything, really, participate in the signaling of disability? What about scenes where I make efforts to be perceptibly deaf, drawing on my assumptions about what others are aware of or attentive to? When do others' perceptions of me make my deafness, alongside other aspects of my body they are poised to recognize as relevant, part of ongoing interactional dynamics? These questions underscore that not all of the ways that disability materializes or matters to everyday encounters are about identity. Disabled and nondisabled people alike are always building and entangling dominant and disabled *dis*-attentions through their lived experiences in the world, although some of these *dis*-attentions are more likely to be amplified, and some will take on greater resonance as they intra-act with various material-discursive configurations.

Hekman's account of disclosure, which draws from Barad's theory of agential realism, alongside Sanchez's account of "doing disability with others" can help reshape an onto-epistemological understanding of disability as an emergent intra-acting phenomenon within discursive-material encounters and ecologies. While Tobin Siebers and Rosemarie Garland-Thomson have offered complex embodiment and misfitting, respectively, as ways to acknowledge mutual change in environments and bodies through their encounters, ultimately, as epistemological figurations, both complex embodiment and misfitting more readily acknowledge changes in disabled people's knowledge and identifications rather than in environments and the material world.[24] Hekman's and Sanchez's terms push toward a fuller account of the movements and permutations of disability in the world, many of which do not inhere on bodies or identifications, but all of which involve intra-acting agencies that produce disability as an emergent phenomenon and reveal its mattering in the world.

Signs and other material-discursive phenomena intra-act with perceptual apparatuses to disclose disability in a range of formulations. For Hekman, disclosure can be understood in reference to "an external reality that is the object of discursive practices,"[25] but not one that is waiting to be discovered. "Rather," she notes, disclosure "is a product of [material, human, more-than-human] agents' interaction in a shared environment with a world that emerges through that interaction."[26] These disclosures shape emerging and dynamic cultural orientations to disability, often alongside forms of collective attention and practices of *dis*-attention. This process—what Sanchez terms "doing disability with others"—contrasts with a perhaps more conventional understanding of disclosure as a one-time revelation of something that is not known to others. At the core of this conventional understanding is a set of what Ellen Samuels terms "fantasies of identification"[27] that persistently suggest that identity is something that can be ascertained from or through the body. Systems of racism, sexism, heterosexism, colonialism, and ableism intertwine in these fantasies to produce compounded effects on particular bodies. "By attempting to produce disability as a stable truth, something that can be revealed in a single exchange," Sanchez argues, "disclosure simultaneously causes us to overly invest in utterances we recognize as such and to fail to register forms of communication that we don't."[28] Fantasies of identification thus put stock in readily legible disclosures while obscuring many other potential signs and sites for materializing disability—precisely the process Friedman describes in explaining how perceptions of bodily materiality produce identifications of male and female bodies within a dominant and normative binary gender system (see chapter 1). The complexity of identity and of disability is subsumed under and reduced to particular signs: the hearing aid, the caption logo, the wheelchair icon.

Scholarship on disability disclosure frequently makes the point that naming or explaining a disability productively is far more complicated than making a one-time announcement or proclamation. As Sanchez writes, a fixation on labels or having the right name for a condition, a disability, a form of complex embodymindment "leave[s] no space for bodies (and our understanding of bodies) to change over time,"[29] not to mention the erasures it enacts of "the role of context and conversational partners in determinations about the presentation of disability, the particularities of the power differentials across which we are always communicating in academic settings, and the complex calculations of probabilities of increased or decreased personal safety (physical, emotional, financial) that shape people's decisions about when, where and how to discuss disability."[30]

In the years that I have been moving with the yellow diamond-shaped "Deaf Person in Area" sign, I have yet to find a better metaphor for this conventional process of disclosure than this sign. I imagine it proclaiming—with an exclamation point or maybe three—"Deaf Person in Area!!!" throughout the neighborhood. This is, indeed, how institutions of all kinds, including universities, schools, hospitals, social service agencies, and government bureaucracies, seem to imagine disclosure. You check off a box or name a medical condition and, well, that's it. Only—as the "Deaf Person in Area" road sign makes laughably apparent—nobody knows what to do upon encountering this sign and (presumably) learning that there is a deaf person in area. And when I say "nobody" I do not just mean those who are not deaf or those who do not have close relationships with deaf people: even those of us with intimate knowledge of deafness, even those of us whose everyday experience of the world involves complex onto-epistemologies of deafness, do not know what this sign is revealing.[31] The sign reveals far more about assumptions of deafness as it circulates in imagination than it does about deafness as it materializes and takes shape in everyday interactional possibility.

The "Deaf Person in Area" sign's agential practices, its disclosures of disability, emerge through its influences on how people move, notice, interact, and engage with it. For instance, drivers might adjust their driving behavior. Or they might think to themselves, "I should request a similar sign for my own neighborhood." They could also, as I do here, wonder about the sign and what it conveys. Each of these reactions is a response to disclosures enacted by the sign as it participates in the emergence of reality. As we live and move in the world, we encounter dominant forms of *dis*-attention that infuse our perceptual apparatuses and influence our conscious and nonconscious determinations of what is "relevant" and "important" to notice. For instance, the sign might tell the story that those in the vicinity of the sign need to be cautioned, warned, about a Deaf Person in Area. At the same time, disabled *dis*-attentions also sneak-snake their way into crip forms of attending that resist practices of able-bodied normativity. Such disabled *dis*-attentions led to my surprised reaction at encountering a sign in my neighborhood, joking with my partner that the sign might be there for me. The joke, however, was predicated upon him recognizing as ridiculous the idea of us asking our city to put up a large yellow "Deaf Person in Area" sign. That many people I have made this joke to have not laughed points to the fact that even among disabled attentional practices, hegemonic waves of *dis*-attention shape what is notice-able and perceive-able. We can again recall Friedman's work on perception and categorization, which stresses both the increased focus on and attention to perceived-to-be relevant information and the dismissal of ambiguous or complicating information (see chapter 1).[32] These processes of perception and categorization amidst dominant and disabled forms of *dis*-attention also point to relations between epistemological and ontological becomings. In critiquing the conventional meanings attached to disclosure, Sanchez suggests that "doing disability with others" may move us toward (differently) generative possibilities, noting particularly the ways that material objects such as wheelchair lights, a "DeafBlind and Badass" button, and a "piss on pity" t-shirt serve as object-beings with which people "do disability." To do disability, then, involves attending to the signs of disability emerging and circulating around us, noticing how and when disability is perceived, cued, and engaged. Our changing perceptual practices across different contexts and at different times contribute to a collective understanding of what meanings are associated with disability. Through such efforts we can actively shape and reshape practices of *dis*-attention.

The materialization of disability in public encounters is shaped by perceptual apparatuses heavily influenced by dominant forms of *dis*-attention that are themselves imbricated with perceptual practices that materialize race, gender, and sexuality. This process of materialization is "frictioned," a word that Aimi Hamraie and Kelly Fritsch use to describe the project of creating access as different kinds of bodies and minds move together in shared space.[33] This friction is perhaps particularly apparent in the ongoing violences that have long been documented by disability-justice activists tracing what happens when Black, Indigenous, and people of color (BIPOC) disabled, queer, and trans people encounter police officers.[34] This violence is supported by material environments as well as implicit and explicit codes that shape behaviors, practices, and ways of moving. Dominant *dis*-attentions inexorably orient to disability as a threatening or dangerous difference, making material, that is, concrete, threats that are amplified and transformed as disability materializes alongside other forms of marginalization.

While I focus on encounters in public spaces, perceptions of disability matter to any interaction where collective and individual modes of attention and *dis*-attention differentially materialize disability. Such interactions teach, through mundane, everyday lived experiences, what disability means and how to orient to it, and they disclose how links are woven (as well as frayed or reinforced) between disability and the stories about disability that emerge.

Signs Disclosing

In analyzing the "Deaf Person in Area" sign, my goal is twofold: to deepen the theory of signs of disability by showing it as enlivening both the material and the discursive aspects of interactions and to show how signs of disability shape everyday perceptions through waves of *dis*-attention that entangle with one another. One wave of *dis*-attention involves mainstream orientations to disability that insistently ignore disabled people's onto-epistemologies. A second wave reveals shifting possibilities and openings through disabled forms of perception. The contradictions and tensions among these waves highlight the importance of realizing new intra-active possibilities for materializing disability, for telling different stories at a time when being disabled in public can be dangerous, particularly for multiply minoritized disabled people. The stories about yellow diamond-shaped signs that I share here are not depictions of just one story; they are accumulations of story, filtered through my repeated interactions around the yellow diamond-shaped sign as I have carried it and watched it circulate around me. They are, again, what Titchkosky terms things that are "say-able" about disability. The "say-able" are commonplace, commonsense, general, assumed-to-be, "just how things are," "natural" observations about the world around us.[35] Where and how do these narratives produce the phenomenon of disability? How do they disclose?

The perception of disability is never straightforward, and I hope to show some ways that recognizing disability is shaped by dominant *dis*-attentions that are readily taken up and circulated in uptakes of the signs' ambiguous disclosures. This ambiguity is important to what is left out or ignored in the stories about these signs. As Friedman observes, "When we do not perceive ambiguous details when focusing or categorizing, it is not because these complicating details are so well accepted that they are taken for granted. Rather, the information inattended in focusing is what is threatening to the coherence of our social categories—and therefore to our sense of mental or social order."[36]

The irony, of course, is that while the disclosures of threat are often claimed to point outward *from* the disabled bodymind so identified, the real danger is to the person whose bodymind is disclosed. These disclosures are both material and discursive: histories of discrimination create real effects on people and influence how they move, interact, and are engaged by others. What people perceive from one another's embodied and enminded presence impacts how they move interactionally. Too, material artifacts and environments actively participate in these interactions. In all of this, discursive histories, language practices, framing, self-presentation, emerging and ongoing relationships, and self- and other-construction play key roles.

The specific "Deaf Person in Area" sign that launched my noticing of yellow diamond-shaped signs of disability disappeared from my neighborhood years ago,[37] but it has maintained an active presence in my academic and personal life. Its presence is supported by the frequency with which I have encountered other yellow (mostly) diamond-shaped signs that name a disability or point to a type of disabled person. The genre of yellow road signs of disability includes a wide range of terms, images, and phrasings. Many are diamond-shaped, some are rectangular, and sometimes there is both a diamond and a rectangle. The collection I am about to engage is partial and idiosyncratic to my own movements and relationships in and with the world. I took many of the photographs in my collection while traveling to academic conferences, visiting college and university campuses, or taking trips with my family. Some were shared with me on Facebook, through text messages, or via email, as friends and colleagues performed their own noticing. Figures 2.9–2.11 present some examples to gesture at some of the range of these signs.

On the more than fifty signs in my collection[38] of this specific yellow caution genre appear the following phrases, many multiple times:

Deaf Person in Area
Deaf Child Area
Deaf Child
Caution Deaf Child in Area
Deaf Pedestrians (with flashing yellow lights above and below the sign)
Watch for Deaf Child
Autistic Child
Autistic Child Area
Autistic Child in Area
Blind Pedestrian X-ing
Blind Ped X-ing
Blind Pedestrian
Vision Impaired Person
Blind
Blind Child
Blind Persons Crossing
Deaf Blind Children X-ing
Caution Deaf Blind Child in Area
Handicap Child
Handicap Child Area

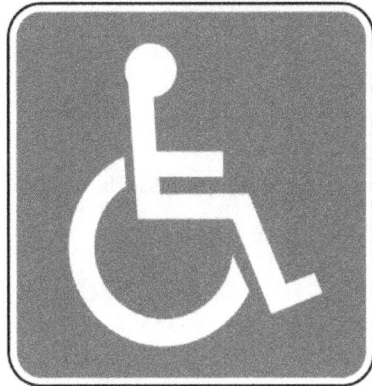

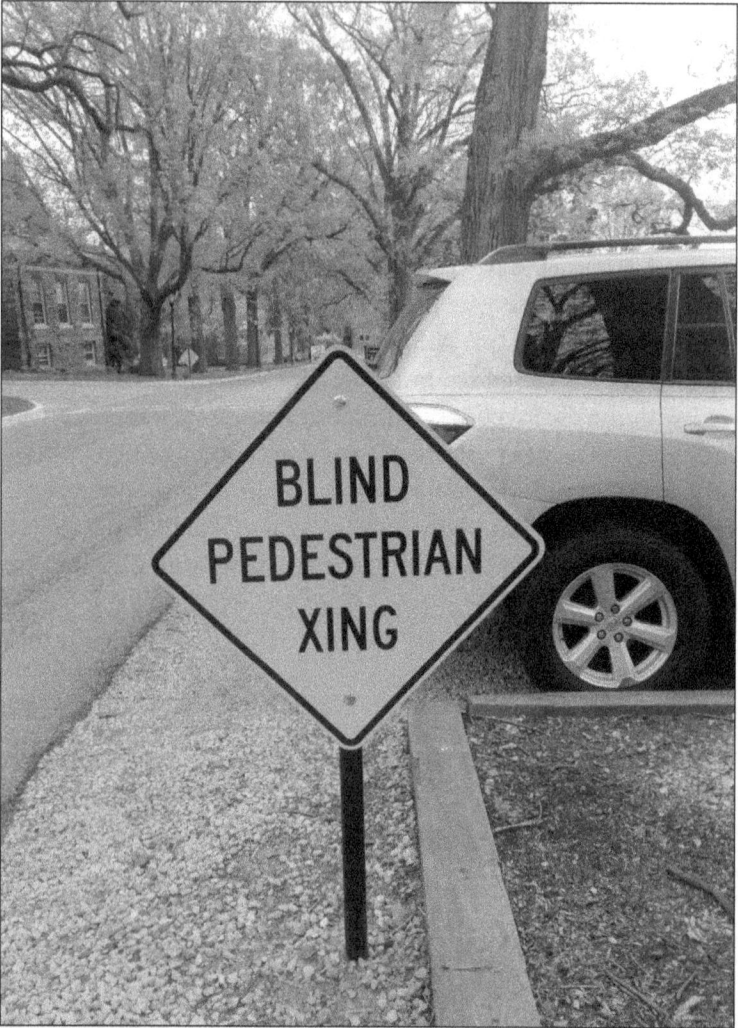

Figure 2.9. Blind Pedestrian Xing. Image description: A yellow diamond-shaped sign that reads "Blind Pedestrian Xing" sprouts from a gravel berm next to a street winding through Haverford College's campus. A car is parked behind the sign. Haverford, Pennsylvania. (Photo credit: Kristin Lindgren.)

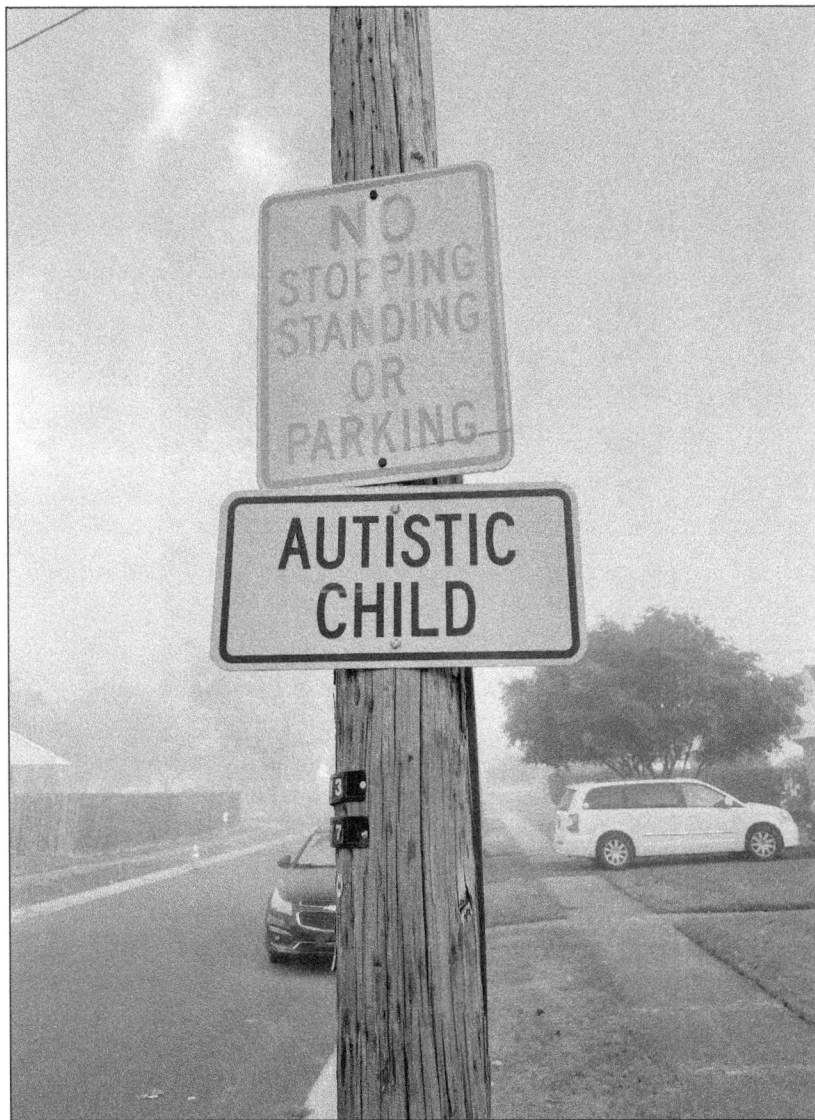

Figure 2.10. Autistic Child. Image description: A yellow rectangle with the words "Autistic Child" is nailed to a telephone pole just below a white "No Stopping Standing or Parking" sign on a city street. Wilmington, Delaware. (Photo Credit: Kaitlyn Delaney.)

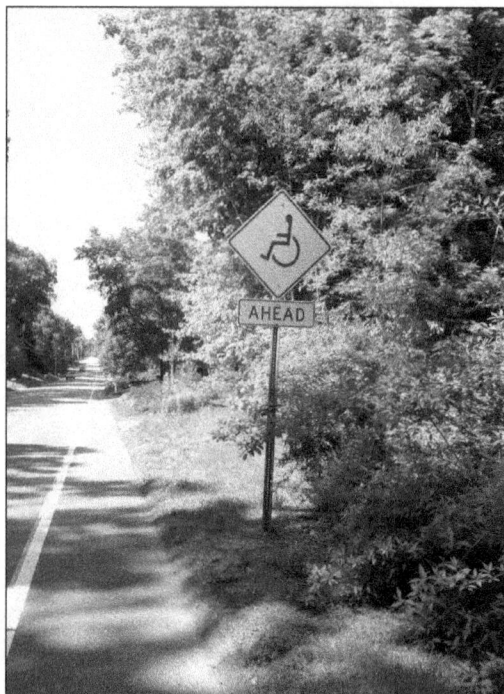

Figure 2.11. Wheelchair Icon Ahead. Image description: A yellow diamond-shaped sign with a wheelchair icon on it and a rectangular sign with the word "Ahead" just below it are planted on a grassy median alongside a rural road. Large, green, leafy trees and bushes fill the side of the road. Ellington, Connecticut. (Photo by author.)

This collection includes a relatively short list of disabilities: deafness, deaf-blindness, blindness, mobility impairments, and autism. Too, in my sample the words "Autistic," "Handicap," and "Deaf Blind" always co-occur with "Child" or "Children." Most of the images I have are from suburban residential developments or along winding rural roads, with only a small number from densely populated and highly trafficked urban settings.

The signs are typically placed by local municipalities, often by specific request from residents with final implementation and decision making performed by city or state Department of Transportation employees. A Google search turns up many examples of online forms, downloadable pdf's and other means by which residents can put in a request for a sign in a specific location.[39] These forms are themselves a genre worthy of further analysis, although they fall outside the focus of this chapter. The behind-the-scenes maneuvers and structures that lead to the placement of a "Deaf Person in Area" sign certainly rely on many forms of *dis*-attention, but my emphasis here is on the interactions that occur once a sign is placed and the stories that emerge as people make sense of the signs.[40]

The Deaf Person in Area Might Not Hear Cars Coming

Perhaps the most common story shared about the sign is, "It's good that there's a sign because the Deaf Person in Area might not be able to hear cars coming." It is commonsense, unquestioned, that this caution is needed because a Deaf Person in Area who (presumably) cannot hear an approaching car might step into the road unexpectedly. As a consequence, motorists need to be vigilant, need to be warned. The sign discloses as valuable and important in order to protect the Deaf Person in Area. *Dis*-attention is central to this story in multiple ways. We do not need an Actual Deaf Person™ for this sign to disclose, and indeed, the sign's disclosures can be understood as relying upon an absent and imagined Deaf Person who needs this sign to disclose for them because their deafness might not otherwise be readily perceptible.

When an Actual Deaf Person™ materializes, multiple forms of *dis*-attention emerge. The ways I *dis*-attend to traffic are sometimes put in tension with the *dis*-appearance of deafness disclosed by the sign. I sometimes respond to this story, then, by mentioning that as an Actual Deaf Person™, I never assume that I can cross the street without looking, that is, without seeking some kind of sensory input that will materialize for me traffic or oncoming vehicles. I tell people that because I know that I will not consistently perceive traffic through auditory input, I always look in other ways. These claims are rarely persuasive, an experience that resonates with Friedman's account of how sensory perception that is ambiguous or that complicates existing frameworks is frequently dismissed rather than folded into a new understanding. And indeed, there are many instances of sensory apparatuses that can misdirect. To take one example, Stephen Kuusisto describes an intersection where the configuration of buildings and the direction of the wind obscure the sound of oncoming traffic such that he cannot rely on sound cues to determine whether it is safe to cross.[41] My interlocutors likewise point out cross-ings with limited visibility (even if they are nowhere near the particular sign[s] under discussion) to argue that you cannot always see a car com-ing. Here my lived experience, my entangled practices of disabled and dominant *dis*-attentions, and my orientations to visual and auditory and tactile sensory input as a white deaf woman are challenged by the sug-gestion that I overrely on sight, and further, that because there are many sounds I do not hear, I do not understand how important these sounds are for safely navigating traffic.

Even should my interlocutor acknowledge the import of my disabled *dis*-attentions, built through a lifetime of carefully visually surveying my surroundings, I am still turned into an exception. They tell me, "well, *you* might look, but Other Deaf People™ would not." This sometimes in-volves the bonus mention of a specific (type of) Deaf Person—real or imagined—who would definitely need protection from the sign. Un-derneath these comments again lurks a disability exceptionalism that casts successful disabled people as exceptions and positions an (often-imagined) other group as those for whom the signs need to exist.[42] Now, of course, my own embodied experiences as a deaf person are not representative of how all deaf people move through the world. And cer-tainly, some of my nondeaf interlocutors have experiences interacting with deaf people that shape how they attend to this sign. But there is something very telling about people who are not deaf assuming that they know what deaf people need in order to move safely through an environ-ment. In this way, as the sign discloses beliefs about the need to hear in order to walk safely around a neighborhood or to follow traffic signals, it also exposes limits of *dis*-attentions that have been shaped through hearing people's perceptual apparatuses. It exposes the limits of hearing people's capacity to understand what it means to not assume that one will hear cars approaching or what it is like to always be vigilant with one's eyes. It also discloses a presumption that the only or primary safety risk here is disability, ignoring the fact that expectations of safety are largely reserved for bodies that are already anticipated within a space.[43]

Indeed, notions about what constitutes safety vary according to not only individuals' disability identification but also their perceptible race and ethnic identification, their gender and sexual identity, their relation-ships in and around an environment, and more. Recent and repeated, persistent differences in how Black and white bodies are treated in public have been made starkly apparent through example after example of Black people being murdered while white bodies are given deference. Thus, we can ask who is likely to believe or assume that a yellow diamond-shaped sign calling attention to a Deaf Person in Area will enhance the safety of said Deaf Person, particularly if the Deaf Person is Black or not read as white. The case of Magdiel Sanchez, a deaf Latino man who was shot and killed by Oklahoma City police even as neighbors and family members shouted to the officers that he was deaf[44] makes such questions deeply pertinent to any exploration of the Deaf Person in Area sign.[45] It is through such questions that the signs disclose presumptions of perceptible embodied privilege.

Not only do my interlocutors generally presume numerous forms of privilege for the Deaf Person in Area; they also draw stark contrasts between hearing *ability* and deaf *inability*. When, for instance, I would point out that in my small college town people regularly walk around with earbuds or large headphones over their ears, I am usually presented with a generous belief in the ability of those people to perfectly apprehend their surroundings. These defenses of hearing ability co-occur with presumptions of deaf inability to move safely through a neighborhood, necessitating the sign. Here again, the sign discloses a persistent cultural orientation to disability as a threat, in this case, to the presumed wholeness of a hearing identity.

Drivers Need to Know about the Deaf Person in Area So That They Will Drive More Carefully

A second common story offered for the "Deaf Person in Area" sign is that "drivers need to know there is a Deaf Person in Area so that they drive more carefully." Instead of centering the Deaf Person in Area's presumed inability to hear, this rationale centers assumptions that drivers may make. If drivers assume that all the pedestrians in their vicinity can hear, they may then expect those pedestrians to stay out of the car's way. Conversely, if those drivers are reminded of a Deaf Person in Area, they may drive more carefully, now expecting that those in the vicinity may not hear a car. Getting drivers to drive more carefully is the focus of many road signs, especially those that feature children (e.g., "Children

Playing"; "Keep Kids Alive, Drive 25"). However, this comment once again assumes that deaf people are not using any other sensory input to try to determine the presence of a car, and it ignores the fact that in the absence of specific guidance, most people do nothing at all to change their driving behaviors.[46] A 2007 Wisconsin Department of Transportation review of existing research argues that "Children at Play" and other warning signs do not change drivers' behavior. The report specifically calls out the intractability of people's belief in the signs' efficacy, noting that "a common theme is the ongoing struggle to explain to members of the public that their requests for these types of signs are based on faulty assumptions about their effectiveness."[47]

One such faulty assumption might be that such signs would not exist without Good Reasons. But Department of Transportation employees, who ultimately construct and place the signs, do not necessarily have expertise around disability. Yellow diamond-shaped road signs that warn about dangerous curves or road conditions may fall squarely within their skill set, but the danger posed by (or to) a Deaf Person in Area is less clearly a topic about which DOT staff can (or should) claim professional expertise. And even when DOT employees may resist placing warning signs, as advocated in the Wisconsin DOT report, residents can (and do) draw on their own personal experiences to challenge the authority conveyed by the DOT.[48] These residents may fear that a driver might not see the Deaf Person in Area or might not drive carefully enough through their neighborhood. Regardless of the process or the human agents involved in the signs' placement, the general perception of the signs' efficacy largely relies on nondisabled people's *dis*-attentions and materializations of disability in public space. Further, these *dis*-attentions rarely account for the entanglements among disability, gender, race and ethnicity, sexuality, and other forms of oppression and/or privilege.

A Deaf Person in Area Might Not Follow Traffic Rules

Finally, a third common rationale is that "a Deaf Person in Area (especially if they are a Deaf Child) might not follow traffic rules." Fears of an accident may be amplified for many parents of disabled children because their children can take longer to learn expected traffic rules and behaviors. As typically framed, the problem is that because of their disabilities, these children may have an especially hard time following traffic rules. This final logic requires some additional parsing. To do that work, we need to zoom out a bit and consider the broader genre of yellow road signs.

The things on yellow diamond-shaped road signs are quite varied and include road hazards (e.g., "Slippery When Wet," "Bridge Ices Before Road"); various areas or spaces (e.g., bus stop; "Rock Slide Area," "Correctional Facility Area"); upcoming road shapes or conditions (e.g., "Lane Ends Merge Left," traffic signal, intersection, sharp curve); vehicles (e.g., fire engine, tractor, bicycle, horse and buggy, school bus); and animals (e.g., deer, alligator, bear, duck, cougar, moose, kangaroo, goose, bison, armadillo, big cat, rattlesnake, cow).[49] The yellow color and (usually) diamond shape associate these signs with warning or caution. Within the broader ecology of yellow road signs, people are not typically indicated. Indeed, the only people I have encountered on yellow caution signs are disabled people, children, and pedestrians, including silhouettes of a running family on a sign posted near an immigration crossing. We might also include here a yellow diamond-shaped sign reading "Correctional Facility Area," which, while not specifically pointing to people, indirectly indexes hitchhikers and blurs the distinction between "Area" and "Person" in that its placement along a road is likely intended to deter motorists from picking up hitchhikers. What do these disclosures reveal?

One way to answer this question is to parallel the common responses to the "Deaf Person in Area" sign with rationales for other things on yellow diamond-shaped signs. For example, one reason we have yellow diamond-shaped signs with different kinds of vehicles on them is that those vehicles move differently than do cars. As a consequence, drivers need to behave differently when one of these vehicles—a fire engine, a bicycle, a horse and buggy, a school bus, a tractor—is in the road. Similarly, being warned of an upcoming change in the road (e.g., a sharp turn or an intersection), a road hazard, or an environmental condition can enable motorists to take appropriate driving measures. All of these things involve caution, encouraging drivers to be attentive to things that they might not otherwise anticipate. These logics overlap significantly with the previous stories about the "Deaf Person in Area" sign.

But then we come to the most varied subcategory of "things that are on yellow diamond-shaped signs": animals. The logics that explain why we have various yellow diamond-shaped signs featuring a deer, alligator, bear, duck, cougar, moose, kangaroo, goose, bison, armadillo, big cat, rattlesnake, or cow in many ways are the same logics that explain why disabled people need to be on the signs. First, there is a presumption that *animals won't follow the rules of the road*, whether this is because they are not cast as intelligent enough or because they are unreliable and unpredictable or because they operate outside the boundaries of human behavior rules. As a consequence, it is drivers who need to be responsible for watching out: they cannot assume that a deer, alligator, bear, etc., etc., in the vicinity will stay out of the way of their vehicle. There is also the argument that *drivers need to know an animal is in the vicinity so they will proceed more carefully*. This argument presents the sign as there for both drivers and animals: drivers will take in the information on the sign—the knowledge that a specific animal is (likely to be) in the area—and adjust accordingly. Therefore, the sign helps support ecosystems that have been disrupted by a thick winding ribbon of asphalt in their midst: if motorists take more care, then the road, the cars, the people, and the animals may be able to coexist.

A third cultural logic also explains why animals appear on yellow diamond-shaped signs. That is, *a threatening animal is in the area and drivers should exercise caution*. All the animals on yellow diamond-shaped signs can be interpreted in terms of threat—whether the threat is to the animals (by a car hitting or running into them) or to a car (a large animal like a deer or moose can damage a vehicle) or to people in the car (an accident can cause injury; some animals can harm humans). This threat also calls into being other types of threats presented by yellow diamond-shaped signs. This is the flip side to the paternalistic narrative of disability centered in the earlier discussion of responses to the "Deaf Person in Area" sign. While we can read the yellow diamond-shaped sign as an invitation to take extra care, perhaps in the spirit of "it takes a village," the choice to convey this need for additional care on a yellow diamond-shaped sign (and not, say, on another color or shape of sign)[50] communicates that these are intended as warnings.

What does it mean to connect disabled people with these other things on yellow diamond-shaped signs? One answer comes through Mel Y. Chen's theorizing of animacy. Chen notes the linguistic definition of animacy as the "quality of liveness, sentience, or human-ness of a noun or noun phrase that has grammatical, often syntactic, consequences"[51] and then uses this concept to show how "the 'animal' is relentlessly recruited as the presumed field of rejection of and for the 'human.'"[52] Chen identifies the stickiness of animal-like properties to some categories of humans through animacy, a move that ultimately separates them from having full humanity while preserving humanity for those who are not-disabled, not-queer, not-female, not-children, not racial and/or ethnic minorities, and so on. It is no coincidence that the logics used to explain why we need animals on yellow diamond-shaped signs overlap with the logics used to explain why disabled people and disabled children need to be on the signs. Because (some kinds of) disabled people as well as (deaf, blind, deaf-blind, and autistic) children are not presumed to have appropriate cognition or behavior or understanding, they need to be warned about. Others around these (disabled) people and (deaf, blind, deaf-blind, and autistic) children need to be reminded of the presence of disability in order to avoid harm to themselves or to others. This dehumanization is achieved by comparing (some kinds of) disabled people and children with nonhuman animals. Chen writes, "The sentience of a noun phrase has linguistic and grammatical consequences, and these consequences are never merely grammatical and linguistic, but also deeply political."[53] The political nature of these yellow diamond-shaped signs comes into focus when we consider the sorts of animacy—that is, the liveliness, movement, and activity—of groups identified on the signs.

I have numerous examples (and variations) of "Blind Child," "Deaf Child," and "Autistic Child." I have numerous examples of "Blind Pedestrian" and "Deaf Pedestrian" as well as blind and deaf "students." I do not have any examples of an "Autistic Pedestrian" sign or an "Autistic Student" or "Autistic Person in Area" sign. Autism, at least within the genre of yellow diamond-shaped signs that I have collected, is only and always attached to children. The question of disabled personhood and subjecthood, then, is limned through the grammar and genre of yellow diamond-shaped signs. Again and again, these yellow diamond-shaped signs confirm Chen's observation that "vivid links, whether live or long-standing, continue to be drawn between immigrants, people of color, laborers and working-class subjects, colonial subjects, women, queer subjects, disabled people, and *animals*, meaning, not the class of creatures that includes humans but quite the converse, the class against which the (often rational) human with inviolate and full subjectivity is defined."[54]

Let us return to the common responses I get when I raise the topic of the yellow diamond-shaped "Deaf Person in Area" sign. The sticky links between disability and animals that I have been discussing are underscored in the observation that people wearing headphones or earbuds may not hear everything in their surroundings. The (surprisingly fierce) defenses I experience of these pedestrians' ability to hear cars coming, paired with claims that a Deaf Person in Area should announce their presence, resonate with the adherence of animacy to Deaf Persons. The dehumanized "Deaf Person" (etc., etc.) is not *presumed* to have competency and agency in the way that the *presumed* perfectly intact, fully human hearing person with headphones does. The fully human person is often akin to Garland-Thomson's concept of the normate, a mythical figure that nobody actually lives up to but that is imagined as embodying and enminding every form of privilege: white, male, cisgendered, able-bodied, heteronormative, wealthy, and so on.[55] When a real figure is revealed, that figure's departure from or relationship to each of these forms of privilege can then become material for dehumanization, for asserting that anything that happens to them is an individual occurrence rather than squarely set within a nexus of intersecting discriminations and patterns of exclusion and violence aimed directly at particular kinds of bodies and minds.

When we recognize that the signs operate according to an animate hierarchy that places adult humans with full sensory capacity at the top, while children, disabled people, and disabled children fall lower down the scale, simultaneously desubjectifying and objectifying them,[56] we can begin to refigure and reshape some of those associations. In *Beasts of Burden*, Sunaura Taylor urges us to reframe animal and disability rhetorics by "acknowledging the violence caused by such histories of dehumanization, while also taking seriously the need to challenge the role the animal has been forced to play within dehumanizing systems and rhetoric."[57] To be understood as something that would be placed on a yellow diamond-shaped caution sign is effectively to have a comparison made between you and other road hazards, between you and other animals that either do not know or will not follow the rules of the road, or between you and things that are dangerous to drivers. We also can identify a hierarchy whereby autism would arguably be placed below deaf and blind because of its consistent association with childhood and its lack of association with the identities of "Pedestrian" or "Student."[58] These associations do not emerge out of thin air. Here we must consider the background, what Chen identifies as the environments or support systems that make these dehumanizations so sticky, so persistent in our cultural attention. For example, as I noted earlier, many of the images of yellow diamond-shaped signs that I have collected are from suburban locations, largely featuring neatly trimmed yards and single-family homes.[59] This might seem to suggest that disability is such an unusual presence within these environs that it needs to be proclaimed by a large yellow sign. Too, it reinforces links between (presumed) whiteness and assumptions around safety, risk, and disability: the regular frequency of news reports of Black people being shot and/or killed by police officers serves as a violent reminder of the kinds of bodyminds that might expect to feel "safe" in being identified and/or pointed to.

The logics of the yellow diamond-shaped signs thus disclose assumptions about disability as inability, disability as threat, and disability as requiring protection. The signs, through dehumanization and objectification of disability, disclose ableist logics that deny agential possibilities for disabled people. As Taylor writes, "Ableism helps construct the systems that render the lives and experiences of both nonhuman animals and disabled humans as less valuable and as discardable, which leads to a variety of oppressions that manifest differently."[60] When we reveal the operations of animacy that play out on yellow diamond-shaped signs, then, rhetoricians and community members can intervene in these structures of meaning making by challenging and addressing the oppressive logics that perpetuate particular *dis*-attentions toward disability, race, gender, class, and more. The point is not simply to critique dehumanization but to "examine the systems that degrade and devalue both animals and disabled people—systems which are built upon, among other things, ableist paradigms of language and cognitive capacity."[61] Such systems serve as persistent sources of oppression, particularly as disability is deployed within various configurations to set entire populations and groups apart from worthiness and value. Our perceptions participate in these oppressions by reinforcing or eroding links between (some kinds of) humans and objects, drawing on processes of dehumanization that separate disability from personhood.

The "Deaf Person in Area" Sign Pushes Back

Thus far in this chapter, I have centered on the yellow diamond-shaped "Deaf Person in Area" sign disclosing, but I now want to conclude by considering how the "Deaf Person in Area" sign, in Hekman's terms, "pushes back, effects the result."[62] Such a consideration means asking, What would it mean to openly invite, even embrace, the links and associations between object beings and human beings? What might it mean to "unbecome human," as Eunjung Kim puts it? Kim suggests that such an enfolding might enable inclusivity while also loosening associations that circumscribe agency and seem to accord agential possibility only to certain kinds of beings.[63]

Scholars working in phenomenology of race, trans studies, and disability studies have insisted on the imbrication of epistemology and ontology as the materiality of particular forms of embodiment participate in possibilities for knowing. Such possibilities emerge out of the particularity of perceptual apparatuses and material arrangements, as the analysis of the yellow diamond-shaped "Deaf Person in Area" sign above suggests. Perceptual apparatuses are likewise shaped by the lived experiences that are often centered in phenomenological accounts even as they always enact inclusions and exclusions. Charles W. Mills identifies one such exclusion in his account of materializing race. He critiques white-centered bodies of theory because they "take for granted as natural the personhood of the humans that are their theoretical units, failing to see that this (recognized) personhood is *itself* a historical product that likewise needs to be denaturalized."[64] How we perceive shapes what we find, always in dynamic relation to the material configurations of our perceptual apparatuses. Recognizing exclusions within our perceptual frames and working to change the conditions for our perception matter to the phenomena that disclose to us.

Within disability studies, an epistemological (or, for some, cripistemological)[65] turn has reinforced the value of disabled ways of knowing and moving for the world. Many of the contributors to a collection of essays on *Deaf Gain*, for instance, invoke ways that deafness as a lived, embodied engagement in the world has value, as epitomized in the collection's titular shift away from "hearing loss" and toward "deaf gain."[66] Collectively, this work underscores that *dis*-attentions shaped by disabled epistemologies are essential for countering harmful *dis*-attentions that elide disability or compartmentalize it into "appropriate" or "acceptable" or "expected" spaces (see chapter 1). My experiences navigating an academic career as well as my material embodiment as white, deaf, and female have shaped where and how I engage as a scholar and an activist. These experiences of complex embodiment have produced, as Siebers would posit, a body of knowledge.[67] But these experiences are questions of *being* and not only of *knowing*. That is, they are ontological.

Ontology is important here because within disability studies, the turn to epistemology has often been a means for reclaiming disabled people's subjecthood and of distinguishing humans from nonhuman animals, so as to reassert disabled people's humanity.[68] However, epistemology is a tenuous—even false—means for suggesting human exceptionalism.[69] The frequency with which many disability communities carve out space for white disabled people without building multiply minoritized coalitions makes pressing the need for arguments rooted in radical inclusion. Such radically inclusive coalitions are centered in Sins Invalid's *Skin, Tooth, and Bone: A Disability Justice Primer;*[70] in Alice Wong's Disability Visibility Project;[71] and in Leah Lakshmi Piepzna-Samarasinha's *Care Work.*[72] The creators of these texts explicitly describe their coalitional work as resisting the systems of oppression that Talila Lewis names in defining ableism. Lewis's definition of ableism, built in communication with other Black and brown disabled activists, recognizes the mutual dependency between ableism and racism, especially anti-Blackness, that exploits bodies for money, profit, exploitation, and resources, only to discard them when they are no longer useful or profitable.[73] To resist these systems of value, then, requires each of us to build perceptual apparatuses that will enable us to perceive phenomena that emerge through these mutually reinforcing oppressions. The challenge for white people, cisgender people, heterosexual people, and nondisabled people, then, is that of refusing the persistent invitations we receive to not-notice and not-attend bodies' mattering. We are often encouraged to push to the background, rather than explicitly surface, our (non)conscious noticings that feed these systems of oppression. As Sara Ahmed puts it, "Whiteness is a straightening device: bodies disappear into the 'sea of whiteness' when they 'line up' with the vertical and horizontal lines of social reproduction." She adds, "Bodies might even 'move up' if they line up, which requires leaving one's body behind."[74] Those of us who experience these forms of privilege, then, are encouraged at every turn to ignore, suppress, minimize, and even deny them. This means needing to work harder to materialize our bodyminds and make them available for noticing as part of our everyday lived experiences.

The imbrications between interlocking systems of oppression and the mutual dependencies between ableism and anti-Blackness can make it challenging to materialize phenomena and enact boundaries amidst these entanglements. If, as Barad suggests, our boundary-drawing practices are never absolute and they "have no finality in the ongoing dynamics of agential intra-activity,"[75] then we have a responsibility to resist dominant *dis*-attentions that perpetuate oppression. Eunjung Kim makes this point when she reminds us that inclusion is never complete or whole, arguing that while objectification is sometimes pointed to as a means of dehumanization, this approach "does not reflect how humans are embodied, attach themselves to objects, live in proximity to objects, and become dis/embodied as objects" and thus "cannot account for the infinite number of ways in which objects create meanings."[76] That people are shaped by their relationships with objects and material environments is also underscored in Kimmerer's story-theorizing (see introduction). Each of these inquiries is part of ongoing boundary-making practices involving all beings in relation to and with one another.

To make a boundary—an agential cut—is to produce a phenomenon through intra-actions between perceptual apparatus and material world. These apparatuses are themselves dynamic intra-acting phenomena intra-acting with emergent material-discursive systems for organizing and sorting and classifying and acknowledging value. To account for the agential work happening more explicitly within an intra-action, then, we need to avoid a fixation on epistemology and "knowing" as the primary means by which perceptual apparatuses are shaped. Not all perceptions are conscious (see chapter 1), and we need the coparticipation of epistemology and ontology to perceive intra-acting phenomena. To this ontological-epistemological imbrication, Barad adds a third term, ethics: "since each intra-action matters, since the possibilities for what the world may become call out in the pause that precedes each breath before a moment comes into being and the world is remade again, because the becoming of the world is a deeply ethical matter."[77] This ethico-onto-epistem-ology refuses any inherent separability between subjects and objects; there is only agential separability enacted through ongoing boundary-definition processes.

As epistemological theories, Siebers's complex embodiment and Garland-Thomson's misfitting each acknowledge that relations with and communities of disabled people matter for individual and collective perceptual apparatuses. To these theories we can usefully add the recognition that what materializes—ontology—takes shape through agential cuts infused by epistemological beings built through ongoing, iterative material-discursive intra-actions. This process is concerned with what mattering comes to matter, what matterings persistently materialize. Such mattering does not inhere in bodies, particular kinds of bodies, acting subjects, passive objects, or humans, or any aspect of the human/more-than-human world, as systems of oppression and discrimination make apparent. We cannot acknowledge this mattering by simply decentering the human or by trying to enact boundaries more firmly around the human both because these boundaries are always shifting and morphing and because notions of humanness are frequently called upon to shore up oppression and disenfranchisement.[78] Instead, there may be utility in turning to the ongoing dynamics of boundary enactments in which disability is disclosed in different, intra-acting ways. This process usefully extends complex embodiment and misfitting to engage ontological agency more fully. Because complex embodiment and misfitting focus so centrally on reflective learning shaped by everyday movements in the world—that is, on humans' and, specifically, disabled humans' forms of knowing as the locus of agential possibility—they do not have as much to say about questions of agential being. A focus on disability that distinguishes (some kinds of) productive knowledges can thus reinforce subject/object distinctions rather than make possible ethical understandings of the ways that we are, as Barad might put it, "*of* the world in its dynamic specificity."[79]

To reveal agency as not a property of intentioned beings but as emergent within intra-action, we can usefully link Barad's agential realism with Marilyn Cooper's theorizing of rhetorical agency through neuro-phenomenological feedback loops. Cooper's work reduces emphasis on conscious or intentioned actions as central to agency, taking seriously the ways that environments and relationships of all kinds participate in making "meaning provided for free," that is, "built up nonconsciously through intra-acting in the world."[80] Within this framework the yellow diamond-shaped "Deaf Person in Area" sign and my own material embodymindment each participate in continual processes of disclosure enacted through boundary-(re)drawing agential cuts in which the world is made and remade again. Entanglements between ontology and epistemology are key here. As I move with and around the "Deaf Person in Area" sign, new disclosures are always emerging and with them, new perspectives, theories, and concepts. Which disclosures do I *dis*-attend, and in what configurations and relations? These questions are of vital importance because, as Barad reminds us, "Meeting each moment, being alive to the possibilities of becoming, is an ethical call,"[81] and it is one that I argue we have not met where disability is concerned.

At this point I want to anticipate a potential critique of my theorizing here. I have forwarded Hekman's and Sanchez's theorizing on disclosure to suggest disclosure (and disability disclosure in particular) as a process of making determinate (some) properties within particular material-discursive configurations as perceptual apparatuses materialize disability. To resist the common practice of linking disability solely with kinds of bodyminds, I have turned to material environments and particularly yellow diamond-shaped signs that index disability, positing that such signs enact disclosures and consequentially shape the emergence of disability as a phenomenon. But I have also developed these arguments by turning to stories that people tell about these signs, a move that may seem to reinscribe a fixation on human epistemology as well as normate ontologies.

So now, I want to switch the terms a bit. The yellow diamond-shaped signs enact disclosures that materialize through stories that circulate and insistently recirculate. In these quotidian, everyday, mundane, iterative, habitual encounters, the signs' disclosures ooze and seep into discourses and practices that take shape around and through and with the signs. The "Deaf Person in Area" sign reveals differential patterns of mattering that largely emphasize nondisabled materializations of disability;

collective perceptual apparatuses that reveal disability as threatening difference; and the obscuring of entangled racial and class materializations in articulations of safety and danger. In so doing, the signs disclose disability, reveal its entanglements, and underscore its shifting and morphing emergence in conjunction with multisensory input and cultural orientations to bodyminds. These disclosures are not human "interpretations": the signs themselves are agential. Following this thread, the analysis above embroiders a call for stories that resist dominant *dis*-attentions and that affirm complex embodiments emerging from disabled attentional practices.

The surround of dominant *dis*-attentions that shape what and how we perceive is a challenge because these *dis*-attentions reify harmful materializations of disability, solidifying and thickening their associations and practices.[82] Missing from these accounts of disability is the tension between discursive constructions and the reality that pushes back. The *dis*-attentions disclosed by the "Deaf Person in Area" sign largely materialize disability through what people already expect or assume. These expected materializations include disability as problem; disability as threat; and disability as individual deficit, the latter of which is apparent in the fact that many of the signs I have collected photographs of seem to point to a single person. But the sign also pushes back. It refuses these perhaps dominant associations or meanings, not only through disabled forms of *dis*-attention revealed in many deaf people's responses but in the sign's own refusal to participate in or resonate with particular *dis*-attentions. In order to tell better stories of disability, then, we need to (re)shape our perceptual apparatuses to materialize disability in ways that push back against harmful *dis*-attentions. In chapter 3, then, I suggest disabling as one process for such reshaping.

3

Disabling

To tell better stories about disability, to resist the dominant *dis*-attentions that infused the stories that shaped the yellow diamond-shaped "Deaf Person in Area" sign, this chapter turns to a research study conducted by disabled faculty with disabled faculty. This study offered the opportunity to engage with and generate stories disclosed through intra-actions among disabled practices of *dis*-attention, a process that I describe in this chapter with the term "disabling." "Disabling" as I use it here refers to resisting dominant and harmful *dis*-attentions to enable generative possibilities for disabled *dis*-attentions to emerge and thrive. In processes of disabling, disability is shaped and reshaped through intra-actions among multiple disabled forms of *dis*-attention. Put another way, disabling is a kind of world making in which phenomena come to be bounded in different ways as disabled *dis*-attentions entangle.

This use of "disabling" follows the way Amy Vidali and Remi Yergeau have each used the term to point to disability's generative potentials, much as Brenda Jo Brueggemann has done in describing disability as enabling insight.[1] As Vidali puts it, disabling is a process that centers disabled perspectives "in order to innovate, include, and transgress expected and exclusionary norms."[2] In their work, Vidali, Yergeau, and Brueggemann each resist articulations of disability and disabling as negative or undesirable, seeking to invite and encourage processes of disabling. Many others have used "disabling" and "disabled" in ways that resonate with this chapter's argument. In fact, one effect that I hope will come of how I am using the words "disabling" and "disabled" as adjectives in this book is to amplify the many ways that these words point to brilliance, ingenuity, and power and to support more entanglements among disabled *dis*-attentions. However, even as I will identify desirable valences around disabling, it is also important to recognize that a project of disabling does not always point in celebratory ways. The point is not for disabling to become unequivocally positive or to always be desirable. Rather, it is for practices of *dis*-attention shaped by disabled onto-epistemologies to push back against reductive and marginalizing forms of disability that emerge through dominant *dis*-attentions.

One way to understand this framework of disabling comes from Julie Avril Minich's call to understand "critical disability studies as methodology."[3] In her essay, Minich notes a tension between the thriving academic enterprise of disability studies and the relentlessly intensifying neoliberal pressures that keep pushing disabled people and multiply marginalized disabled people out of academia. To understand this tension—and to resist it—Minich forwards a critical disability-studies methodology that would focus on "the social norms that define particular attributes as impairments, as well as the social conditions that concentrate stigmatized attributes in particular populations."[4] These social norms and social conditions participate in the work of disabling as social processes and material realities also shape the emergence of disability as a phenomenon. In a response to Minich's essay, Jina B. Kim offers an example of this methodology as she takes up Alexis Pauline Gumbs's essay "The Shape of My Impact" to forward a "crip-of-color critique." Gumbs's essay describes how leading Black women scholars, including herself, Audre Lorde, and June Jordan, experienced institutional denials of needed support as they faced significant health crises. In the face of these denials, Gumbs affirms women of color academics' refusal to "equate productivity and work with one's life worth."[5] In turn, Kim argues that approaching disability as methodology is "to take seriously this politics of refusal, to recognize disablement and racism as inextricably entangled, and to enact intellectual practices—like resistance to hyperproductivity—that honor disabled embodiment and history."[6] Much like Eunjung Kim's project of "unbecoming human" (see also chapter 2), processes of disabling center intra-acting disabled *dis*-attentions and recognize their imbrication in systems of racism and other interlocking oppressions in ways that create new conditions of possibility for radical inclusion.[7]

When I first started my faculty career, I actively cultivated dominant *dis*-attentions that elided disability: just as I did not want my disability to matter (see introduction), I wanted to prove to others that it should not matter to them, either. I also worried about being left out, negatively evaluated, or excluded from opportunities if I did not smooth others' access to me by making my disability as imperceptible and unproblematic as possible. That these fears primarily related to my deafness, and to a lesser extent my gender, while race and sexuality were more often backgrounded in my active awareness materially shaped my own disabled *dis*-attentions as I made these access decisions. My emphasis on deafness and gender also influenced how disability took shape through my own perceptual apparatus, leading me to recognize some *dis*-attentions and forms of disability while eliding others. There were significant risks in encouraging dominant *dis*-attentions, however. Failing to notice ways that my experience of disability within institutional spaces was smoothed by whiteness and heteronormativity constrained possibilities for building radically inclusive professional spaces. Too, if others around me were not taught to *dis*-attend differently, to resist dominant *dis*-attentions, then my efforts to support my own accessibility could be—and often were—wasted when others would make last-minute changes to meeting venues, modes of participation, or interactional dynamics.[8]

Over time, given the regularity with which behaviors emerging from dominant *dis*-attentions upended my access efforts, I came to realize that my long-term professional success depended on ensuring that others around me could perceive disability and learn from disabled *dis*-attentions. Consequently, I have made efforts—in different ways at different times and in different places—to support disability perceptibility as well as to encourage others to incorporate disability into their everyday practices of noticing. This work often involves investing in longitudinal relationships that support knowledge building around disability, and it is one of the reasons my scholar-in-residence experience at Michigan (see chapter 1) was so jarring: I had spent more than a decade at Delaware building these relationships and working toward relative predictability regarding accommodation and access, and it was daunting to start that process again in an even more hostile environment for disability.

While many of the *dis*-attentions that I experienced at Michigan also characterized my early years at Delaware,[9] by fall 2019, when I took the scholar-in-residence position at Michigan, a relatively straightforward process for requesting interpreting was in place at UD, and I could generally expect that Delaware's centralized Disability Support Services would be able to accommodate my requests. Too, if there were problems with interpreting availability, I had other strategies I could deploy, and some of my colleagues had come to recognize their own responsibility for thinking about access in ways that did not put all of the labor on my shoulders. But getting to this point had required me to educate a revolving door of department chairs (four in my first five years at Delaware) who were charged with evaluating my performance as a tenure-track faculty member but none of whom, prior to meeting me, understood how the lack of reliable access to high-quality interpreting services mattered to my work. It required me as well to negotiate with scores of staff members and colleagues to educate them on the importance of securing skilled interpreters who could meet my particular needs.[10]

As I have participated in efforts to support my own and others' experiences of access throughout my career, I have never done this work entirely alone. Sign language interpreters and access providers routinely share their expertise and knowledge with staff members and colleagues. A network of deaf and disabled academics, connected via email, Facebook groups, and various virtual and in-person get-togethers, regularly provides a means for building what Aimi Hamraie calls "access knowledge." Access knowledge, as Hamraie defines it, is "a regime of legibility and illegibility" around "what users need, how their bodies function, how they interact with space, and what kinds of people are likely to be in the world."[11] Access knowledge is at the heart of the crip world building and support that Leah Lakshmi Piepzna-Samarasinha describes in writing about "disabled mutual aid," which, she writes, conjures up "a million examples of subtle, diverse forms of disabled survival work, but which is mostly not seen as 'real work.'"[12] This learning and collaboration with other deaf and disabled academics in spaces where our disabled *dis*-attentions entangle with one another has been an essential element of my persistence in academia.

The process of *disabling* is to resist dominant *dis*-attentions and build different practices of *dis*-attention through entangled disabled onto-epistemologies. In this sense, disabling involves what Hamraie terms "epistemic activism," in which people use their knowledge and expertise to "transform access knowledge from within"[13] as disabled people live, learn, and work together. Such transformations come as disabled onto-epistemologies intra-act and shape disability's emergence within complex environments. When Teresa Blankmeyer Burke shared with a group of fellow deaf academics a form letter she used for communicating her interpreting needs, her language and choice making materially influenced numerous other deaf colleagues who used her letter as a template to create their own.[14] Blankmeyer Burke's entire website, in fact, exemplifies the kind of knowledge-building and relational work deaf academics often undertake in navigating sign language interpreting accommodations. Too, friendships with deaf academics across the United States have led me to new ways of noticing and paying attention to deafness as well as to how whiteness shapes my experience of deafness and disability. These colleagues showed my deafness back to me in ways markedly different from the encounters I had with nondeaf members of the university communities I lived and worked in, and these disabling encounters led to shifts in how I navigated my everyday environments.[15]

Such shifts have a long history in disability scholarship and activism, and they often germinate in environments created by and for disabled people. In addition to the accounts of epistemic activism that Hamraie traces in *Building Access*, disability activists have worked to cultivate the brilliance and ingenuity that emerge as communities of disabled people work together and share expertise. Piepzna-Samarasinha, drawing on decades of work by disability activists, describes "care webs" built among predominantly people of color and queer and trans disabled people "attempting to dream ways to access care deeply, in a way where we are in control, joyful, building community, loved, giving, and receiving, that doesn't burn anyone out or abuse or underpay anyone in the process."[16] In like fashion, Alice Wong's Disability Visibility Project[17] amplifies stories about disability that center on multiply marginalized disabled creators, activists, artists, and scholars all working to forward new ways of understanding disability. In contrast to the collective and mutually reinforcing crip environments and interactions that Hamraie, Wong, and Piepzna-Samarasinha describe, my experiences as a white disabled academic at predominantly white campuses and in overwhelmingly white professional organizations suffused with cultures of eliteness, perfectionism, and hyperability have involved continually challenging misconceptions, resisting stereotypes, navigating disability-related microaggressions that are simultaneously raced and gendered, and repeatedly explaining why I needed people to change their behavior. But

I did catch glimpses of disabled community building when I spent time among disabled academics at conferences, during writing retreats, and in visits to one another's homes. In these encounters, we did not spend our time proving to one another how we were disabled or defending our needs for particular ways of moving. The way my body came to differently relax in these interactions taught me to *dis*-attend differently, to *disable.*

I illustrate some of the challenges and possibilities in processes of disabling in the remainder of this chapter by turning to a research interview I conducted with Tonia (a pseudonym), who identified herself as a Black research scientist at an elite, predominantly white US institution who had a chronic lung condition, was immunosuppressed, and had recently undergone a double lung transplant.[18] Early in our interview, I asked Tonia if she discusses her disability at work. She responded with "Um::, yes, I mean, because my disability is obvious (1.2), um well I guess (1.8), actually, can I rephrase this."[19] This comment is an emblem of the dynamism of processes of disabling and how disability becomes available for noticing. It also indicates how perception and material reality coparticipate in making the world. Note in particular Tonia's pauses, which are significant because, as Karen Barad suggests in *Meeting the Universe Halfway*, "the possibilities for what the world may become call out in the pause that precedes each breath before a moment comes into being and the world is remade again."[20] Tonia lives in a world where her disability is both obvious and not obvious, and these possibilities differently become and take on meaning as the research interview in which she is participating unfolds. Tonia's "obvious" and her shift to "actually, can I rephrase this" thus make and remake the world, bringing possibilities into being, shaping and reshaping them. This is the work of disabling, a process that emerges through lived experience, material encounters, and intra-actions among forms of *dis*-attention.

A significant way disabling happens is through story. To tell a story is to make an agential cut, to give definition to phenomena through intra-action, to enact disclosures. Agency here involves continual movement toward new intra-acting possibilities, often by reconfiguring, reconstructing, deconstructing, or reorienting perceptual apparatuses. As material-discursive artifacts, narratives both produce and make available for examination attentional practices and perceptual orientations that frequently operate outside of conscious awareness. We often do not know what we are noticing until we try to describe or account for those things in story.[21] As Tonia told stories of various experiences during her interview with me, she asserted disability while linking it to Blackness, womanhood, and disability in ways that her colleagues persistently failed to recognize but that she encouraged me—and by extension, readers of this book—to notice. Such links were made possible not only by Tonia's storytelling but also by the material conditions that supported her telling: the interview context and the research and recording apparatus surrounding it.

Engaging with the disclosures enacted by Tonia's narratives can help others disable their perceptual apparatuses. Importantly, disabling is not an automatic process. As many of the stories already shared in this book make apparent, disabling does not launch immediately upon encountering disability in some way, shape, or form, whether on a yellow diamond-shaped sign, in a literary or cultural text, or in a world suffused with ideas and discourses about disability. Rather, it is a process whereby the perception of disability—the intra-action between sensory input and perceptual apparatus that materializes disability as a phenomenon—is shaped and (re)shaped through ethical engagement. We can observe such ethical engagement in modes of interaction that productively support attention to disability, such as those described by Hamraie, Piepzna-Samarasinha, Wong, and many others who have written about coalitional and crip community building and collective access. These disabling encounters attend to the ways that disability matters and is consequential for the world's becoming, and they open up possibilities for understanding disability that are often foreclosed by dominant practices of *dis*-attention.

Unlike the stories suffused with ableist *dis*-attentions discussed in chapter 2, the stories Tonia related emerge within an interaction actively shaped by multiple disabled onto-epistemologies. To show this disabling at work, I linger both with the stories Tonia shared during her interview and with my experiences learning to do academic research. Our interview context is an intra-acting participant in materializing phenomena, and the materiality of the interview context as well as of the recording and analytic tools that made it possible for me to work with Tonia's narratives are part of disability's emergence. For this reason, I begin by describing the design, implementation, and analytic procedures of this research study through the framework of disabling to stress how much it matters who researchers are, how the research proceeds, and how research intra-actions unfold.

Disabling Research Design

When Tonia declared that her disability is obvious and then corrected herself, she was making her disability available for perception to an interviewer interested in her experience of faculty life and disability. At the same time, she was describing her experience of making disability perceptible in her workplace. How she came to tell this story at this particular time was shaped as much by the design of the research project that led us to share time together on the phone as it was by her lived experiences of navigating disability. Between 2013 and 2016, I collaborated on an interview study focused on disabled faculty members' experiences with disability disclosure in professional contexts. During study recruitment, more than one hundred potential interviewees indicated their willingness to participate by completing a ten-question demographic survey in which they identified their academic field, institution and institution type, faculty position and rank, identifications around race, gender, sexuality, and disability, and preferred contact information and interview modalities.[22] Interviewees were selected over a three-year period with the aim of including as many different types of experiences and identifications as possible. At the end of my involvement in the project, I had conducted seventeen interviews using a range of interview modalities and practices:

- in-person conversation in sign language;
- in-person spoken conversation;
- in-person spoken conversation using a sign language interpreter;
- telephone conversation using an Internet relay;
- telephone conversation with a sign language interpreter;
- signed conversation over videoconference;
- spoken conversation over videoconference;
- asynchronous email exchanges; and
- synchronous instant-message conversation.[23]

In intentionally incorporating distinct communicative modalities for conducting interviews, this study cut against some orthodoxies in research methodology, particularly where consistency across interview experiences is concerned. This choice was motivated by principles of inclusion and accessibility as well as an approach to interdependent research developed by Margaret Price[24] that recognizes that in order for disabled faculty to participate in a research study, they need to know that their needs around communication access will be met.

When Tonia volunteered for the study, she had already encountered multiple signs of disability that may have disclosed to her the centrality of disability to this project. For instance, the study's recruitment email pointed to disability in its subject heading and description of the project, and the demographic survey that all study volunteers completed asked after their preferred communicative modes. Additional signs of disability potentially emerged in the recruitment email's reference to "accessible interviews,"[25] a term that invokes but is not limited to disability-focused forms of access. Such acknowledgments that study volunteers would have needs and references to how those needs might be considered in designing research interactions likely influenced participants' willingness to volunteer for a research study.

As rhetorical and persuasive encounters, interactions during study recruitment are consequential for the stories and data that may be generated, a point that Ellen Barton stresses in an analysis of two case studies of medical-study recruitment. As Barton notes, because recruitment "decision making takes place between real people, in real time, in (semi-)ordinary language that is typically more indirect than direct, within complex situations that are institutional and symmetrical,"[26] it therefore has ethical and persuasive dimensions that merit rhetorical consideration. Signaling disability is one such rhetorical element. However, such signaling is complex, and how disability materializes is affected by myriad entangled, intra-acting phenomena. For instance, despite my own commitment to negotiating accessible communicative contexts for both myself and those I interviewed, it was still challenging to interpret potential signs of disability taking shape from my intra-actions with the information participants provided in the demographic survey. While the survey asked after participants' disability identification as well as their preferred modalities for an interview, this naming, much like the "Deaf

Person in Area" sign (see chapter 2), did not necessarily convey information about the kinds of interactional patterns that would be most useful or accessible during an interview.

Even when people identify their preferred modes of communication, those needs and preferences are likely contingent on dynamic and emerging ecologies in which intra-actions unfold. Just as my experiences of trying to smooth others' access to me could be upended by shifts in the interactional context, this too was a possibility for these interviews. Each interview involved at least two disabled people learning to interact together in shared social space. This was a sometimes-fraught process whereby interviewers and interviewees had to work together to navigate the best ways for those encounters to proceed. While I went into the interview process anticipating that I would take interviewees' preferences into account, I did not to the same degree consider what information interviewees might interpret about me that would influence their decisions about how to move in this study. These are disabling processes as disability comes to be identified through complex intra-actions that simultaneously shape as well as close off possibilities.

Let me share one example of this kind of disabling. Participants were able to select "sign language" as a choice of modality for an interview. But the survey provided no information about how a signed interview might proceed. Would the researchers be working with interpreters? Would the participants have a choice of interpreters to use for the interview? Do the researchers themselves know sign language? If yes, how well do the researchers communicate, expressively and receptively, in sign language? None of these questions were answered in the recruitment survey itself, and answers to them would have almost certainly mattered to potential participants thinking about whether they would, in fact, be willing to participate in a signed interview. Relatedly, I did not explicitly name my gender or my racial identification in the recruitment email or demographic survey. This of course does not mean that study volunteers had no concept of my race or gender given how central these identifications are to everyday interaction. My name, which in the United States is typically read as female, was shared in multiple places. Because I did not—in these early encounters and emails—explicitly mark a gender identification, indicate my preferred pronouns, or name my racial identification, given patterns whereby dominant identities tend to remain unmarked,[27] this unmarking may have led participants to assume normative identifications on my part, potentially perceiving me as white and female. Too, the recruitment email included my email signature, which had a link to my faculty website as well as to the website for the "Disability Disclosure in/and Higher Education Conference" that I co-organized in the fall of 2013. In this way, the recruitment email made available (some) messages about (some) identifications, including whether I explicitly marked them or left them unmarked. What researchers assume can go without saying, and what needs to be made explicit in study recruitment are significant questions, especially for people from underrepresented or marginalized communities who may be making decisions about volunteering or continuing with research projects, both for the participant's (emotional, mental, and/or physical) safety and because of long histories of exploitation of people and communities by academic researchers. At this point, now that I have set the stage for Tonia's interview, let us listen to some of her stories.

Disabling Narratives

Tonia narrated a career trajectory that began at her elite university in a tenure-track faculty position. When the institution's and her colleagues' productivity and work expectations proved to be unsustainable in concert with the effort that it took for her to maintain her health, an experience aligned with many accounts of Black women's overwork and institutional refusals to accommodate,[28] she took a less intensive but still demanding research position. After her double lung transplant, she made yet another transition, from full-time to part-time employment. These changes in her physical health, her employment status, and the obviousness of her disability to others around her led her to narrate disability in several different ways over the course of the interview.[29] When she began her position, she was able to manage her chronic lung condition without using external oxygen, so few of her colleagues knew about her health issues. Once she needed oxygen (either carrying a small portable tank or using a larger tank that stayed in her office), her health and disability became more readily perceptible by others. And when she no longer needed oxygen after her transplant, others' attention to and perception of her disability again shifted dramatically.

Tonia's stories[30] repeatedly expressed how hard it was for her to make disability available for noticing within her workplace despite the severity and significance of her disabling condition. This difficulty contrasted with the ease with which disability was recognized in our interview interaction. I opened our interview by asking her to describe her job and her disability, and she began by referencing the Americans with Disabilities Act: "Um, so I have uh::: (0.5), I guess, I have a (1.0), disability in (1.2), activities of basic living as in I can't breathe on my own."[31] She named limitations placed on her daily activities by her chronic lung disease: "It's hard to move around, I'm limited in how much I can carry, I'm limited in how fast I can move (1.2)."[32] She also referenced multiple health conditions that required intensive management, including not only her chronic lung disease but also transplant recovery, cancer, and complications associated with cancer treatment. This list might suggest that Tonia's disability would be readily apparent to others around her, given all that she was dealing with and her shifting levels of physical functioning. However, the opposite was the case, as Tonia's stories—the narrated events—repeatedly reinforced instead her colleagues' refusal to recognize disability, denials that closed down possibilities for Tonia's survival and well-being. At the same time, our interview together—the storytelling event—participated in the process of disabling, of making disability available for noticing through intra-actions among disabled experiences and perceptual apparatuses.

At multiple points in our interview, Tonia illustrated her colleagues' and her institution's refusal to acknowledge her disability by invoking her oxygen tank, which often served as a metonym for her disability. As a material artifact, the oxygen tank was complexly entangled with sociomaterial arrangements, embodied realities, and practices of perception. The oxygen tank's shifting perceptibility, alongside Tonia's material embodiment in her workplace environment, points to what Moya Bailey has termed "misogynoir": "the uniquely co-constitutive racialized and sexist violence that befalls Black women as a result of their simultaneous and interlocking oppression at the intersection of racial and gender marginalization."[33] According to Bailey, while the harms caused by misogynoir impact nearly every aspect of Black women's lives, its effects are particularly evident in its impact on their health, given that "the stress and material consequences of systemic oppression make it nearly impossible to have physical, mental, and social well-being in a white supremacist patriarchal country."[34] Tonia's stories and her practices of disabling emerge in these intersections among Blackness, womanhood, and disability.

Multiple processes of disabling unfolded through Tonia's interview and her narratives. To understand how Tonia's stories participated in disabling processes, it is useful to note the distinction that Stanton Wortham, drawing on Roman Jakobson, makes between what he calls the narrated event and the storytelling event. For Wortham, the narrated event is "the event described by the utterance," while the storytelling event refers to "the interactional context within which the speaker utters something."[35] The narrated events that Tonia described included accounts of moments when others harmfully *dis*-attended—that is, ignored or elided—the effects of Tonia's chronic lung condition as well as moments when she cultivated productive practices of *dis*-attention that could enable her colleagues to materialize disability and support her persistence at work. These efforts to materialize disability were entangled with the ways that Tonia's race, gender, and institutional status were available for her and her colleagues to notice.

Tonia described these narrated events in a particular material-discursive context that also shapes narrative emergence: the storytelling event. Thus, intra-actions over the course of the storytelling event matter to how stories emerge. A second layer of disabling, then, involves the interview interaction during which Tonia and I perceived aspects of each other's embodiment and their mattering to our encounter. Tonia and I each made and remade ourselves over the course of the interview encounter, revealing and reshaping disability. Recall the discussion of perception in chapter 1 in which sensory input passes through a perceptual apparatus, producing an intra-action that is itself shaped by myriad forms of disabled and dominant *dis*-attentions. These intra-actions enact agential cuts that give definition to particular properties or characteristics of phenomena (including disability), making some determinate while leaving others indeterminate. It is in this chaotic dance of determinate and indeterminate, of boundary (re)drawing, that disabling happens in the course of the world's everyday mattering.

To illustrate some of these entanglements as well as the ways that the interview context supported and participated in Tonia's telling, I turn to a segment of the interview titled "Do You Discuss Your Disability at Work," after the question that spurred the stories within it. Several forms of disability perceptibility and signs of disability, largely centered on the presence or absence of the oxygen tank, emerged across the eleven narrative episodes in this segment, which totaled 143 lines of transcript. Tonia began by saying, "When I took the job, I already had the lung disease, that was debilitating, but people didn't <u>know</u>."[36] But, she explained, this imperceptibility shifted because "once I needed oxygen (1.5), obviously everyone knew."[37] Transcript 3.1, titled "Materializing Disability at Different Times," shows the final three narratives of this segment. In narrative 9, Tonia describes the general state of things post-transplant when she no longer needed to carry oxygen with her. In narrative 10, she relates a specific encounter with a colleague whose question about Tonia's health elided Tonia's embodied presence. And in narrative 11, she recalled a moment when her boss explicitly denied her disability. The narrative and temporal slippages across these accounts are important to understanding disabling, as past experiences commingle and participate in present ones. In reading these stories, pay attention to how Tonia describes her disability and its perceptibility to those around her. Note, too, that the interpreter and the signed mode through which I access Tonia's words in real time are absent from this transcript, an important methodological issue that I will return to later in the chapter.

In these segments, Tonia attaches her disability perceptibility to the tank: when the tank was present, disability was potentially perceptible; when the tank disappeared, so, too, did her experience of disability, at least in others' perceptions. In turn, these narratives illustrate some of the challenges around materializing disability, challenges that may be amplified within contexts like Tonia's elite, predominantly white institution that are suffused with dominant *dis*-attentions that actively maintain a distance from disability. This distancing enables those around Tonia to ignore, elide, or suppress attention to her disability. While Tonia regularly referenced the figure of the oxygen tank (e.g., "once I needed oxygen [1.5], obviously everyone knew") she also noted that her disabling condition was more readily acknowledged by staff members than by the faculty colleagues featured in the narratives above. As she put it, "Our clinical staff members (1.0), would only, you know, they might ask me

Narrative 9: After Transplant It Was Harder

66	TONIA	um:: (0.5)
67	STEPH	right
68	TONIA	and
69		then after transplant (2.5)
70		it was harder
71		because (1.8)
72		people (0.5)
73		just think you return to normal (1.0)
74		and they didn't really underst[and
75	STEPH	[right
76	TONIA	um:
77		why
78		I wasn't back at work full time
79	STEPH	right
80	TONIA	um::
81		or (1.3)
82		why (0.5)
83		you know like why
84		I could get sick so easily

Narrative 10: The Co-Leader of My Group Asked "Is This Really Serious"

85	TONIA	and um
86		actually I'm even on a leave of absence at the moment
87		because I'm going through rejection from my transplant
88		and to give an example
89		[um
90	STEPH	[oh jeez
91	TONIA	I had when I explained to (1.0)
92		my

(continued)

Narrative 10: The Co-Leader of My Group Asked "Is This Really Serious"

93		like
94		the co-leader of my group
95		that I would [need to go out=
96	STEPH	[mh-hmm
97	TONIA	=because I was rejecting my lungs (0.8)
98		her response was
99		is this really serious (1.6)
100	STEPH	oh my go[sh
101	TONIA	[and
102		and I was like (1.0)
103		ri[ght=
104	STEPH	[um
105	TONIA	=okay::
106		um
107		so
108		you know
109		and and again
110		she's like nonclinical staff but
111		it blows my mind (1.0)
112		that (1.0)
113		that's the kind of
114		response I was getting
115		and I'm like
116		[you know=
117	STEPH	[right
118	TONIA	=I can't breathe
119		and that [I'm=
120	STEPH	[right
121	TONIA	=losing lung function rapidly
122		and ((chuckles)) (2.4)

Narrative 11: My Boss Said to Me, "Oh You're Not Disabled"		
123	TONIA	so (1.5)
124		you know I feel like I've always been up front
125		with it but I think that
126		even though I've
127		been up front with it (1.5)
128		peopl::e
129		as my boss said to me
130		she's like
131		oh
132		you're not disabled (1.0)
133		um (1.4)
134		[she's like=
135	STEPH	[mhhh
136	TONIA	=I don't consider you disabled
137		and I'm like
138		I need oxygen
139		Like
140		what else do you need (1.4)
141	STEPH	right
142	TONIA	you know
143	STEPH	right

how I was feeling today, but they would only discuss it with me, if I brought it up, with, them,"[38] and "our other staff members quite freely (1.2), would comment."[39]

As a material object that took shape both as a larger tank that lived in her office and as a smaller portable tank that accompanied her outside of her office, Tonia's oxygen tank is a polyvalent sign of disability that matters to her interactions with others. But the tank alone does not materialize disability, and different perceptual apparatuses can erase or subsume possibilities for disability's materialization. In particular, medicalized frames do not always overlap with and in fact, frequently emerge in complex relationship to disability. Narrative 9 reveals a generic account (describing a habitual state of things) as Tonia explains that "people (0.5), just think you return to normal (1.0)" (lines 72–73). In narrative 10, Tonia offers an episodic account exemplifying this generic perception, relating an encounter during which she communicated to her group coleader that she would need to take a leave because of post-transplant rejection and to which the coleader responded by asking, "Is this really serious" (line 99). Tonia's reaction was one of shock: "It blows my mind (1.0), that (1.0), that's the kind of, response I was getting, and I'm like, you <u>know</u>, . . . I can't <u>breathe</u>, and that I'm, . . . losing lung function rapidly" (lines 111–21). The assumption that her breathing issues were obvious, perhaps especially so because she was "losing lung function rapidly," was belied by her group coleader's question. When I followed up, asking how Tonia responded to this encounter with her group coleader, Tonia explained, "I think I was too:, I didn't respond, I was too dumb struck (0.7), like (0.5), that, she even <u>said</u> it."[40] The episodes in transcript 3.1 thus reveal ways that each of the characters—the generic "people" in narrative 9, Tonia's group coleader and boss in narratives 10 and 11, and Tonia in her responses to each of these scenes—are all employing different perceptual apparatuses with regard to the oxygen tank and Tonia's embodied presence. And in her telling, Tonia works to enable my access as an interviewer to some of the signs of disability she displays as well as to others' perceptions of them.

These distinct observational apparatuses make different agential cuts and differently materialize disability as a phenomenon and differently participate in processes of disabling. Consequently, obviousness is not always, in fact, obvious. To understand why this is the case, we can return to Asia Friedman's articulation of perceptual filtering (chapter 1), in which observers selectively attend to particular details deemed relevant, while filtering out those assumed to be irrelevant or unimportant. The accounts of perceptual filtering that Tonia described and that Friedman theorizes around gender perceptibility resonate with phenomenological work on the perception of racial embodiment. Linda Martín Alcoff draws on Maurice Merleau-Ponty's work to note that racial perception relies upon often-backgrounded racial structures—"the field, rather than that which stands out"—resulting in a situation where "perceptual practices involved in racializations are then tacit, almost hidden from view, and thus almost immune from critical reflection."[41]

Merleau-Ponty describes such perceptions in terms of habit, rather than conscious attention. As Alcoff explains, because habitual perception is so unconscious, "interpretation is the wrong word here: we are simply perceiving."[42] Sara Ahmed puts it this way: "When something becomes part of the habitual, it ceases to be an object of perception: it is simply put to work."[43] Such unconscious, habitual perceptions can function as what Daniel Kahneman has described in terms of "fast thinking,"[44] and as what Charles Mills has forwarded as an account of racial embodiment in which "the social ontology of a racialized body politic becomes incarnated in the material bodies of its members, fleshed out in their reactive behaviors, [and] incorporated in their perceptions and conceptions."[45] Habitual thinking, then, matters to the narrated events Tonia describes as her colleagues enact perceptual apparatuses that treat some details of her embodiment as relevant for noticing, enact meaningful boundaries around race and disability, and elide some details as irrelevant or nonsignificant. It matters too in the storytelling event as I make my own perceptions as a disabled white woman interviewer working with a white woman interpreter to interact with Tonia on the phone as she shares her stories.

The Narrated Event

When I asked Tonia to describe some of the ways that people around her might notice her disability, she named a number of multisensory means by which disability—primarily her breathing issues and chronic lung condition—can be perceptible to others: she wears a nasal cannula that people can see on her face; she carries oxygen with her in a tank or as a liquid; she is often out of breath (something that others can see or maybe hear); and if she is wearing a pulse flow oxygen machine, the pulses of air make noise. She also alludes to other forms of disability perceptibility, such as when she describes strategies she uses to negotiate meeting times and locations as well as her use of a scooter. This list in no way suggests the full range of means by which Tonia's disability can be perceptible to those around her, but it does convey some that she readily cues into as potential signs of disability. Not surprisingly, visual perception dominates this list, and many of the things she names are medical accoutrements. This medical link is important not only because of the impacts of misogynoir that Bailey documents but also because, as Bailey and Izetta Mobley point out, "equity for queer, trans, and Black people also has been overwhelmingly about access to adequate medical care," which in turn "requires a complex and nuanced engagement with the medical needs and realities of some populations."[46] Within this medical frame, signs of disability emerge through intra-actions among sensory input, perceptual apparatuses, and phenomena as agential cuts make and remake boundaries around disability. Here, boundary-making processes involve medicalized frames that entangle with but do not always constitute disability and that themselves are imbricated with racism, sexism, and misogynoir.[47] These representational messages infuse everyday encounters through practices of *dis*-attention that encourage attention in some ways and discourage it in others.

To understand how boundaries delineating what was—and was not—disability came to be enacted as Tonia narrated her colleagues' perceptions of her, let us revisit narratives 10 and 11 from transcript 3.1. In both narratives, people who are higher up in Tonia's workplace hierarchy deny or dismiss the presence of disability despite perceptual evidence to the contrary. Considered one way, these interactions reveal the influence of ableist *dis*-attentions, and they point to the threat that disability might pose to the status of working at this elite institution and/or to a researcher identity. Bailey draws on Alcoff's work to point out that racism depends on perceptible difference "to determine which bodies are expendable," adding that this perceptibility then means that "in this cultural moment of Black hypervisibility, Black women are particularly vulnerable."[48] Tonia wants—needs—her colleagues to recognize the severity of her health issues and their disabling effects. She wants them to disable her. Being recognized as disabled would enable her to access the health care she needs as well as to be affirmed and supported in taking a leave (with the hope of eventually returning to work).

Instead, Tonia's claims to disability are swept aside with her group coleader's "is this really serious" (line 99) as well as her boss's casual "I don't consider you disabled" (line 136). Her boss may intend her comment as a compliment, a distancing of Tonia from disability because she is exceptionally good at her job or because she succeeds beyond expectations. However, as Allison Hitt argues, these "rhetorics of overcoming," which she defines as "discourses promoting the idea that disabled [people] must overcome their disabilities in order to be successful, to fit in, or to meet the standard" ultimately do more to make nondisabled people feel better about disability than they do to support what disabled people might need.[49] Indeed, notwithstanding its backhanded compliment, this denial effectively ensures that Tonia's colleagues will not make any changes or adaptations that might enable her to persist at work.[50] While her group coleader did not refuse association with disability, she nevertheless enacted a refusal to perceive disability. In neither acknowledging nor affirming Tonia's need to take a leave, her question instead put additional emotional and access labor[51] on Tonia's shoulders as Tonia worked to make her chronic lung condition perceptible as disability. When I asked Tonia how she responded to the group coleader, she described being "too dumb struck (0.7)" to say anything in the moment: "I just, you know, ranted to my friends." But she also went on to explain that she later worked to consider her group coleader's position too, realizing that at the moment of the encounter she had not "had enough time to: (1.5), remember that other people are going through their own things (0.5), so, and I just, you know, try to tell myself well (0.5), there've been a lot of times that I've been sick, that they have said, this is serious that (1.5), °it°, you know it is serious . . . and I, you know, I try, I just try to remember that it's very tiring to be a caregiver, or to be the coworker of (0.6), someone (0.5), that is (0.5), constantly going through this (0.8)."[52]

This emotional labor—whereby Tonia is acutely conscious of the work others are undertaking and weighing and considering their emotional needs even as she manages her own emotions and needs in the face of a life-threatening illness and her desire to keep working at a job she loves and excels at—only added to Tonia's experience of access fatigue. Too, Tonia was being worn down not only with demands for access labor but with repeated microaggressions at the intersections of race, gender, and disability.

Indeed, securing accommodations through recognition of her disability was, for Tonia just as for the Black feminist academics Gumbs writes about, literally a matter of life or death. At one point in the interview, Tonia referred back to the conversation with her boss represented in transcript 3.1 and explained that that conversation occurred two weeks before she went on leave. "And I was just like, I'm just sitting here in your office out of breath, because I walked here (0.5), trying to make our meeting time (0.6), and you, . . . don't consider me, disabled (1.0), and I was like, well the ADA considers me disabled."[53] Whether observers cue in to Tonia's health issue or her disability (or something else entirely) depends on the perceptual apparatus that they enact in that intra-action. Recall Barad's discussion of the distinction between uncertainty and indeterminacy (see chapter 1), which states that measurement—in this case, Tonia's presence intra-acting with an observer's perceptual apparatus and the emergent agential cuts and boundary definition—creates particular configurations that materialize phenomena. The phenomena do not exist prior to their emergence through agential cuts enacted during intra-action.[54] What this means for Tonia is that for most observers, Tonia's breathing and/or her oxygen tank cannot simultaneously be insignificant, a matter for casual small talk, *and* deeply meaningful, an indicator of a serious and life-threatening disabling condition. Her oxygen tank and her breathing patterns are not incidental happenings. At the same time, they are evacuated of significance: just an oxygen tank; just some difficulty breathing. Materializing both can only be achieved by toggling between different orientations to the scene, much like the familiar optical illusion showing either two faces or a vase, but not both simultaneously.[55] When Tonia's breathing patterns and oxygen tank disclose "a health issue," they are available for discussion and notice-*able*. But when her breathing patterns and oxygen tank might disclose "disability" instead, they are subsumed by forces of *dis*-attention. Far from being just a matter of different terms for the same thing, the difference between whether her colleagues materialized a health issue or a disability was deeply consequential. These terms reflected emergent outcomes of intra-actions between the perceptual apparatuses that Tonia and her colleagues are poised and ready to deploy in order to access—that is, observe—Tonia's presence.

The Storytelling Event

I have been unpacking Tonia's interview narratives for the ways that characters in the narrated events enacted disability perceptibility. I now want to consider how Tonia and I materialized disability within the storytelling event. As I listened and responded to Tonia's stories during our interview, I was drawing on the information that Tonia

shared in the study's demographic survey alongside what I was perceiving during our conversation while also learning about her material
embodiment through the stories she shared. Tonia's colleagues almost
certainly attended to her racial and gender self-presentations and physical embodiment, but I did not experience these self-presentations in the
ways I am most accustomed to through our phone conversation. While
the demographic survey asked after various identifications, during the
interview I only asked Tonia to explicitly describe her disability perceptibility and did not likewise ask her to describe her race and gender
perceptibility. This makes challenging a fuller accounting of the ways
that Tonia's disability perceptibility is shaped by the materiality of her
raced and gendered embodiment. Both Tonia's disability and her racial
mattering were dynamic and always-changing processes of boundary
definition and redefinition as we intra-acted together. The materiality
of my experiences with these identity categories and how they shape my
practices of *dis*-attention is thus an important participant in the emergence of Tonia's stories.

In the case of Tonia's interview, the similarities and differences that
I perceived among our identifications and embodiments mattered to
how I responded to her accounts and asked follow-up and clarifying
questions. Throughout, I cued an orientation to disability and signaled
awareness of many aspects of disabled experiences that are not recognized in the everyday interactions Tonia narrated. This interactional
cueing shaped Tonia's accounts in that she did not have to do more to
make her experience of disability perceptible to me as an interviewer.
I accepted from the start that this was an account of disability, cueing
that emerges in transcript 3.1 through my continual backchannel utterances such as "right" (lines 75, 79, 120, 141, 143), as well as in the evalu-
ations I offer on Tonia's experiences, as when I said, "oh jeez" (line 90)
after Tonia mentioned she was experiencing transplant rejection and
"oh my gosh" (line 100) when Tonia related her group coleader's question. Tonia's stories here were invited, given shape, and supported by
an interactional context that involved disabled onto-epistemologies and
acknowledged—sought out—disability from the outset. One clue that
Tonia picked up on these cues comes through her use of "you know,"
which she said five times across these three stories (lines 83, 108, 116,
124, 142). "You know" is an example of what Deborah Schiffrin calls

a discourse marker,[56] and as such, it can serve several important discursive functions: it can serve as "a marker of meta-knowledge about what speaker and hearer share" as well as "a marker of meta-knowledge about what is generally known."[57] "You know" thus works as a check-in to confirm that speaker and audience share knowledge that can enable the storying and conversation to proceed. In Tonia's account, then, she was checking in with me to ensure that I understood the significance of these stories, that I was following along.[58] These interactional dynamics participated in the interview's unfolding, including intra-actions among forms of *dis*-attention and relationships to disability that make disability available for perception, that *disable*.

Tonia's stories were disabled through her participation in an interview with a disabled researcher who was interested in stories about disability from faculty members who identify as disabled. That such audiences for research about disability are relatively rare matters for the knowledge that is built about disability within myriad multi- and interdisciplinary academic fields. Most disabled people who participate in research have their stories told by nondisabled researchers who may have varying relationships to disability in their own lives, ranging from living with or growing up with disabled family members to experiencing aging and age-related declines in function that can sometimes be read as disability to being disabled themselves.

Disabling in Tonia's interview is a process that not only involves explicit identifications with disability but also requires perceptual apparatuses attuned to race, Blackness, womanism, and misogynoir. I have at times wondered how this interview might have unfolded differently—with different stories and different boundary making—with a disabled Black woman researcher. In asking this question, I am not suggesting that only people who share identifications should coparticipate in research interviews together. My experiences interviewing have underscored many ways that my own race, gender, and disability identifications matter in these contexts. Sometimes shared identifications enabled productive questions and possibilities to emerge, while in other cases they led me to presume commonality of experience when it might have been beneficial for me to practice more detachment. Rather than centering on shared identification, instead, we can learn from Sami Schalk and Jina B. Kim as they describe feminist-of-color disability studies and assert it as "a critical methodology and political category that can be taken up by scholars and activists of any gender or racial identity."[59] Tonia's storying is an entangled process whereby intra-acting phenomena emerge and come to be bounded through perceptual apparatuses. These apparatuses are built through lived experience, in the ways that bodies are read and responded to in the world, and in their material encounters across numerous spheres. Both Tonia and I bring these apparatuses to bear on the unfolding interview. In engaging with Tonia's stories as a white researcher, I recognize I have a lot of (un)learning to do when it comes to understanding the centrality of race to my perceptions of disability, given that at every turn white people are encouraged to not-notice race, to background it, and to ignore the structures that support so many of our easy movements within environments. Whiteness is, as Ahmed puts it, "a bad habit."[60] Schalk and Kim's words are a reminder of the ethical responsibilities of knowledge production as Tonia and I engaged together. They call upon me to recognize how my habits and practices have been influenced by research traditions replete with "unacknowledged whiteness" and to instead center feminist-of-color scholarship to transform how disability comes to be perceived.

While many interviewing textbooks suggest the value of interviewers being relatively detached recipients of interviewee narratives so as not to overly influence the telling and the stories that are ultimately shared,[61] it is nevertheless important to remember that complete detachment is not possible. As my questions around the mattering of race and womanhood above indicate, even when interviewers are asking after events or phenomena they have not personally experienced, that detachment is still doing interactional work that matters to the stories that get told. Storytellers are always working to figure out who it is they are talking to and to understand what kind of audience is receiving the narratives they are telling. That interactional work is consequential for the knowledge that emerges within an interview.[62] If we begin from this baseline, then it is even more essential for academic research and knowledge production to become radically inclusive. In Tonia's interview, for instance, she told stories about her experience with disability that built on what she assumed regarding what I as an interviewer (already) know about disability; she did not have to explain disability from scratch. That it is unusual in many research contexts for disability as a phenomenon to emerge from entanglements among multiple forms of disabled *dis*-attentions, as happened in Tonia's interview, speaks to the importance of disabling knowledge by designing research projects in which disabled forms of *dis*-attention intra-act. Creating generative conditions for disabling, however, can be exceptionally hard, a point to which I will turn in the next section.

Disabling Research Apparatuses

The challenges Tonia narrated of materializing disability in everyday interactions with her colleagues were inflected by her professional status as well as cultures of whiteness and eliteness that actively maintain separations between faculty and disability. Tema Okun, in collaboration with others, has identified numerous properties of what they name "White supremacy culture," including "perfectionism," "defensiveness," and "only one right way."[63] When I read Okun's description of these features in a handout aimed at supporting workplace cultures in transforming them, I felt viscerally the ways in which I had willingly—even eagerly—internalized and embraced these properties as I worked on this study as a researcher with access needs. Despite the many ways that the study's interdependent methodology[64] pushed me to recognize the mattering of my disability, race, and gender more openly in the ways that I conducted research and generated knowledge, I still resisted taking this mattering into account. I repeatedly resisted *disabling* my research process. To give one example of this resistance, for most of the data-generation period, I refused to entertain the suggestion that I could request sign language interpreting for some of the interviews I was arranging.[65] Throughout this study I needed prodding to take seriously the mattering of how I navigate communication access. The mattering of my access needs is particularly evident in the work it took for Tonia and I to be synchronously present for a spoken conversation on the phone. When I conducted two phone interviews early in the data-generation process, I used an Internet relay because I did not want to use interpreters (see introduction). At the time, I explained this choice as simply personal preference and, if I am honest, mostly tried not to think about it too much. It took me a long time to recognize—much less openly admit—that questions about why I was so resistant to using an interpreter in these situations were legitimate ones.

One explanation for my resistance may be rooted in what Yergeau describes as a persistent assumption that disabled people are designed for but never the designers. As Yergeau explains, this assumption "positions disabled people as passive recipients. It creates an us/them divide between the able-bodied savior-designers and the disabled victim-users."[66] To request interpreting in this framework would mean identifying as a "disabled victim-user" rather than as the designer and active agent in a research study—a move that cut against the grain of institutional cultures of whiteness and white supremacy that routinely displayed perfectionism and defensiveness and almost never invited vulnerability or acknowledgment of needs. These dynamics shaped me as I navigated everyday lived experience and as I moved in concert, and even tension, with other disabled people. Dominant *dis*-attentions seeped into my researcher identity through my persistent sense that my access needs were less important than those of the participants, as well as in the suggestion that perhaps, if I could not flex and bend to all of my participants' needs, I should not be doing this kind of research. Such sentiments were amplified by the ways that elite and predominantly white workplace environments regularly discouraged attention to researchers' bodyminds, to their race, disability, and gender identifications, and to their vulnerabilities.

These cultures of perfectionism and individualism also led me to resist exposing my experiences of access to others' scrutiny. I worried, What if doing research interviews with an interpreter made people feel less confident in my ability to do research? What if it led them to disqualify my interpretations? And as I have written this book, I have probed more deeply my readiness in some ways and my naivete in others for conducting the kind of study I hoped to do. For instance, just as I note about hyper-able researchers, my own dominant identities—as a white cisgender woman in a heterosexual partnership—have enabled my access to particular opportunities but have also required me to build accountability and humility in recognizing the limits of my own perceptual apparatuses and the possibilities that might emerge from various research intra-actions.

The process of recognizing how cultures of white supremacy and dominant *dis*-attentions shaped my involvement in research was especially fraught in my negotiations around sign language interpreting during interviews for this study. I ultimately conducted three interviews for which I requested sign language interpreting, all near the end of my data generation for this project. Multiple factors affected my decision to make these accommodation requests: (1) several interviewees' selection of telephone as a preferred interview modality; (2) the impossibility of attempting phone interviews without some kind of access; (3) my dissatisfaction with the accuracy and timing of the Internet relay service I had tried early in the study; and (4) that I had worked with my department and my university's disability services office to build an interpreting apparatus that enabled me to fully participate in teleconferences. As my story at the start of this chapter might indicate, that last consideration was years in the making.

Over my career, I have learned to carefully assess when and how to make access requests. When I suspected it would involve significant effort to build a successful apparatus for my participation, I had to weigh the time and energy it would take to build that apparatus with the (longer-term) value such an apparatus might have for me. Too, I always made these kinds of decisions against a backdrop of access fatigue, the constant accumulation of demands for my time and energy in ensuring my own access.[67] While I arrived at UD in 2008, it was not until 2012 that I made the effort to figure out how to work with sign language interpreters in order for me to be present during phone calls. That experience helped me learn what did and did not work in these settings as well as how best to arrange the material surround to ensure my participation and access. Not only did I need to have regular experiences with particular material configurations involving the conference telephone and the department's conference room, but it was also important for me to have working relationships with specific interpreters whose skills were a good fit for my preferences and needs. My willingness to make efforts to secure my own access to research interviews in this study was thus shaped by my familiarity with my institution and particular accommodation structures, ongoing lived experiences and practices of *dis*-attention, and institutional support from my department chair and accessibility providers as well as UD's Disability Support Services office.

This example of regularly requesting interpreting amidst workplace cultures of white supremacy, dominant *dis*-attentions, and highly gendered norms and practices shows how much who I am as a researcher matters to the interview experience in its material unfolding.[68] My onto-epistemology in its complex becoming involves not only my experience of disability, race, and gender but also how I come to understand the ways that others perceive me and navigate my material presences. Just as I will always have to work to unlearn whiteness and actively notice the effects of my white body as I navigate institutional spaces,[69] I will also always have to work to unlearn dominant ways of *dis*-attending that perpetuate ableism, anti-Blackness, and misogynoir and continue to build new, disabled *dis*-attentions that resist white-supremacist cultures. Such efforts are shaped by the materials of and environments for research. Here, then, I want to take up the mattering of apparatuses for generating and analyzing data.

Sign Language Interpreting as Material-Discursive Research Apparatus

Because my interview with Tonia took place over the phone and was facilitated using sign language interpreting for me, a deaf interviewer, it involved a research apparatus that included me, an interpreter, a conference phone, a video camera, chairs for me and the interpreter to sit in, and a table. Figure 3.1 is a screenshot from the video of this interview and shows a conference room with two people seated at a round table— the interviewer, me, a white woman wearing a sleeveless dress and scarf, and an interpreter, a white woman wearing a cardigan and knit shirt. My gaze is focused on the interpreter, whose hands are held up midsign. A conference phone and paper and pen are on the table.

In the case of Tonia's interview, the sign language interpreter changed my access to the recorded data. When the recording only includes spoken language and no visual complement or faces that are too small or blurry for me to effectively employ speech reading, I depend on the time stamps embedded in Transana, the analytic software I chose to help me navigate and sync written transcripts with video data. The local graduate students who generated rough transcriptions of the interview data inserted time stamps as they transcribed,[70] and these time stamps enabled me to navigate to particular points in the transcript or the video. Because none of the transcribers I hired for this project knew sign language, they

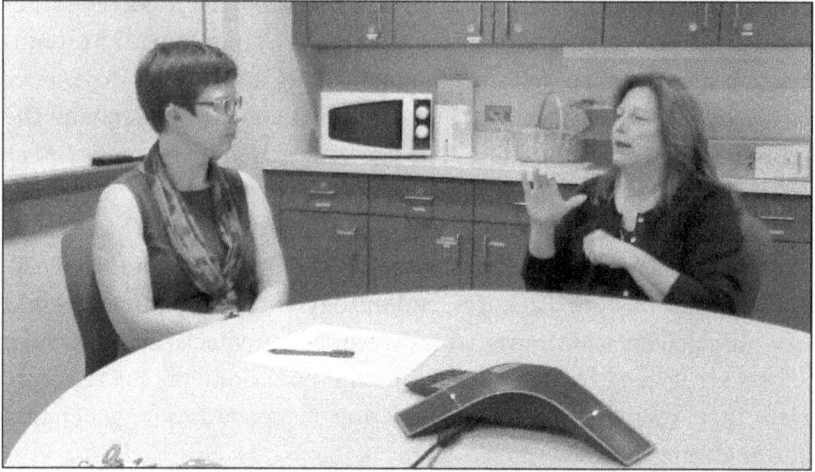

Figure 3.1. Screenshot of interview scene captured on video. Image Description: a conference room, with cabinets and a counter with a microwave, a basket, and a cardboard box in the background. In the foreground is a round table holding a conference phone, some paper, and a pen. Two people are seated at the table: the interviewer, a white woman wearing a sleeveless dress and a scarf, and a sign language interpreter, a white woman wearing a cardigan and knit shirt. The interpreter's hands are frozen midsign and the interviewer's gaze is focused on the interpreter.

listened only to the audio data and did not attend to the interpreter's transliteration. When an interpreter was on screen, however, I could navigate through the video recordings in Transana with ease and ready comprehension even without an external transcript or embedded time stamps. In other words, when an interpreter was on screen my relationship to the audio and video data was fundamentally transformed. Despite this dramatic shift in my experience with the data as well as the thought I have given to transcription practices, it took me years to recognize that I was completely eliding the interpreter's role in this process. In fact, I was well into the drafting of this book when an early reader of this manuscript explicitly asked me to think about the role of translation, interpretation, and the interpreter's presence as an integral part of the mattering that shaped the emergent narratives. This invitation once again required me to confront the dominant *dis*-attentions that, at every turn, encouraged me to ignore my own experiences of disability.[71]

Given this recognition of the interpreter's role in processes of disabling, some readers may be surprised that transcript 3.1 does not reveal any hints of the signed modality through which I accessed this interaction in real time. Indeed, none of the interview transcripts—even those conducted fully in sign language—include a systematic method for sign language transcription that would enable me to attend to the interviews' ongoing interactional unfolding in the same ways that I can with oral data. In working with sound data, I have a long(er) tradition of transcription practices and conventions to draw upon in systematically representing participants' utterances-in-interaction.[72] There is no similar tradition, or even shared systematic approach, for transcribing sign language interaction. Consequently, disabling is not just about the way that my interaction with Tonia shaped the stories that emerged during data generation but is also about the processes by which disabled researchers intra-act with and transform the materials and environments of research.

In "Inclusion, Sign Language, and Qualitative Research Interviewing," I wrestle at length with these questions.[73] While signed interviews were easier for me to navigate, I also found that there were no readily available means for moving signed interactions into written forms, much less written ones that would enable the kind of interactional analyses that have long been the focus of my work. These challenges, along with feelings of fear and vulnerability around nonnormative interviewing techniques, contributed to the elision of the sign language interpreter and sign language modality that enabled my access to Tonia's interview scene both during data generation and during analysis. And yet, that choice, to not-transcribe the interpreter, to not-account for her participation in this scene, is consequential for the emergent analysis as well as for our understanding of the materiality of narrative itself. I need to continue to disable my research, to more fully affirm and recognize the role of disability and its mattering to how I generate knowledge.

Working toward this kind of disabling also requires attention to the imbrication of race, gender, and sexuality with disability's emergence: because these categories fundamentally change how disability comes to be perceived and materialize, they are essential to understanding disabling, disclosing, and *dis*-attending. Tonia's accounts described practices of *dis*-attention that persistently elided innumerable cues conveyed by her material presence, practices learned and cultivated within environments that perpetuate misogynoir.[74] To understand this, we cannot only ask after Tonia's identification with disability: those listening and engaging with her stories must also understand how they are perceiving race and gender. What material, environmental, and/or discursive cues are pointing to disability, to race, to gender? How do these cues intersect and intra-act with perceptual apparatuses? What perceptual apparatuses participate in disability's emergence? What cues for disability, race, gender, sexuality, are different people encouraged—and not encouraged—to notice or pay attention to? There is no ready checklist, but some questions important to adding to our interview repertoires might include explicitly inviting participants to name—and describe—identifications that matter to them and their experiences, and for researchers to attend to what they display and make available about themselves for participants to understand the research context. What aspects of the interview context and environment enable embodied and material perception? What are the consequences and implications of particular research apparatuses for generating knowledge and intra-acting with research participants? These questions can help begin processes of disabling research, work that must involve disabled *dis*-attentions intra-acting to (re)shape the knowledge that emerges. In the next chapter I turn to considering how knowledge generated through research gets dispersed and becomes available for various forms of perception as academics and writers navigate mainstream currents of *dis*-attention in moving their work toward publication.

4

Dispersing

While on a junior faculty sabbatical in 2012 and completing the manuscript of my first book, I developed a vampire-like schedule in which, after tucking my kids into bed, I headed to my basement office and wrote through the night. When my family—my husband and my then four- and two-year-old children—woke up, I would come upstairs and hang out with them as they ate breakfast. After they left the house to start their day, I would head to bed, where I would read for a bit before falling asleep. The books I read that spring were ones that had been repeatedly called to my attention by the disability studies scholars who made their conference presentations accessible to me (see introduction). Those early mornings, holding books in my hands while snuggled among pillows and blankets, marked for me the start of a serious engagement with disability studies that went beyond building academic friendships and involved reshaping and materializing disability in all aspects of my life.

The experiences and decisions that led a stack of disability memoirs to be propped up along the wall by my bed are part of a complex process of textual emergence and dispersal. The story of dispersing that I want to tell in this chapter involves numerous entangled intra-acting processes that include recommendation cycles, learning whom to listen to, deciphering and imagining audiences, encountering audiences and (re)shaping our conceptions of them, and the surprising and mundane work of accumulating expertise and knowledge through lived experiences. The concept of dispersing extends this book's conceptual vocabulary for signs of disability by considering how textual production and shifting contexts participate in materializing disability and enabling its perception. While chapter 2 focused on environments suffused with ableist *dis*-attentions, and chapter 3 considered the imbrication of onto-epistem-ologies centered (in different ways) on disability, here I trace the diffraction effects created by different waves of *dis*-attention.

"Diffraction" is a term that describes how waves behave when they encounter obstacles. For instance, when two pebbles are dropped into a pond at the same time, when the resulting ripples meet, they produce diffraction patterns, showing interference points where the ripples reshape one another. Any time waves encounter other waves or an object, or move through an opening, diffraction occurs, such as when sound waves blast from different speakers, when ocean waves crash against a rock, or when light waves move through window blinds. If we approach *dis*-attention through diffraction, then we can begin to notice how different waves of *dis*-attention meet and interfere with one another, consequently (re)shaping the world-making possibilities in any given intra-action. Various forms of reshaping through diffraction undergird this chapter's work on dispersal. With the concept of dispersing, I extend the discussion of narrative and materiality to consider disability's emergence through processes of entextualization, the process of moving (often spoken) discourse into another (often written) context, thus enabling that discourse to circulate differently.[1]

One form of entextualization involves moving the habitual experiences I had while writing my first book into the stories shared in this book. These experiences, far from being just mundane, easily forgettable, everyday encounters, have been essential for producing the book you are now reading. The vampiric routine I settled into during that sabbatical ten years ago contributed to my choosing to read disability memoirs. They were texts I could hold in my hands and read in a relaxed fashion. They were also relatively affordable, available in paperback and on the used book market, and reading them shaped my perceptual apparatus for noticing disability and my understanding of what disability could mean and be. These books—Eli Clare's *Exile and Pride*, John Hockenberry's *Moving Violations*, Harriet McBryde Johnson's *Too Late to Die Young*, Simi Linton's *Claiming Disability*, and Nancy Mairs's *Waist-High in the World*[2]—were published in the late 1990s and early 2000s and were all written by white disabled people with generally readily identifiable disability experiences. I read them as a white deaf woman on the tenure track writing a book about the negotiation of difference in writing classrooms. While I was still uncertain about the role that disability studies would play in my thinking and writing and did not see this early-morning reading as central to my book project, I did want a better understanding of conversations I had been eavesdropping on for years. My own and these authors' race, gender, and disability identifications shaped both my perceptual apparatus for noticing disability and how disability emerged for me.

Scenes like the ones above—of reading in bed, of the texture and weight of particular kinds of books, of how books came to be stacked up in particular areas of my house, or of what motivated me to pick up this book or that one—are not regularly written into scholarly narratives.[3] Notwithstanding their mundanity or the challenges involved in perceiving them, material intra-actions involving researchers' lived experiences are central to the world-making possibilities of disabling. I became aware of this dynamic early in my career when I began having recurring in-person encounters with people who asked me to account for my body in my writing. These requests contrasted with my observation that it was not conventional for many of the academics I was reading to write into their scholarship physical descriptions of their bodies or self-presentations. This realization speaks to the relative homogeneity of the scholarship I was reading, given that scholars whose bodies and minds push against expectations regularly and often do write their bodyminds into their work. The differences between what was available for noticing as people interact with me in various ways and what I make explicitly available in my writing motivated my first disability studies publication. That article, titled "On Rhetorical Agency and Disclosing Disability in Academic Writing," begins by narrating several scenes in which audiences engaging with my written scholarship solicited explicit recognition of my embodiment and my experiences with disability. The persistence and accumulation of these encounters disclosed to me my own disability, forged in relation with others as various practices of *dis*-attention intra-acted in these scenes. Over time, as I came across different audiences—readers of my work, editors and peer reviewers, conversational interlocutors, conference and lecture audiences—I learned strategies for seeking out and building the audiences that would most support my research and thinking. This sometimes meant interacting with specific people, encounters that were made possible and shaped by each of our bodyminds, while at other times it required me to imagine audiences different from the ones I encountered in my daily life. Such work also required me to push back against and resist centering mainstream or normative audiences.[4]

In the account above, I have stressed how everyday habitual experiences enculturated and encouraged various practices of *dis*-attention as I engaged disability studies scholarship, disability memoirs, and my own work in the field. I have also pointed to the centrality of imagination for shaping *dis*-attention. The link between imagination and everyday experience recalls the work of Asia Friedman and Eviatar Zerubavel (see chapter 1) as they explain that what we perceive is shaped by what we expect, leading us to notice what we look for.[5] As Tanya Titchkosky puts it in terms of disability, "We imagine disability in a variety of ways, and when we notice it, we imagine that the image we notice is, indeed, disability."[6] As an integral aspect of many forms of *dis*-attention, imagination actively participates in disability's emergence. Imagination can both elide and ignore ambiguous or contradictory details as well as resist such erasures, particularly around the intersections of race and disability. Remember that Friedman's work on gender perception stressed a binary conception of gender not because such a perception is "correct" but because it was what interviewees reported. In turn, "what unavoidably remains *unnoticed*," Friedman explains, "are the evidence and details that would support other perceptions and categorizations—and by extension other social worlds, organized around different rules of relevance."[7] In *Bodyminds Reimagined*, Sami Schalk shows how Black speculative fiction creates new imaginative possibilities by stretching and revising ideas about race, gender, and disability. As Schalk writes, while autobiographical and biographical work portraying disabled lives as well as realist fictional accounts have long been recognized for the ways that they resist "limited, problematic, or oppressive representations of marginalized people," such challenges "can also occur through speculative fiction, through nonrealist, fantastical, and nonhuman contexts that change the rules of reality, making us think more critically about how our current rules and assumptions about (dis)ability, race, and gender have come into being in the first place."[8] Imaginatively cultivating disabled *dis*-attentions is likewise significant to Josh Lukin's theorizing of what he terms "recognition," a reaction he describes as a textual encounter that leads him to "say 'Oboy, this names a thing I recognize: I am in a world where others experience it.'"[9] Like Schalk, Lukin develops his account of textual recognition from his engagement with nonrealist science fiction as he points to the role that texts play as they disclose and take active roles in the making of meaning and the mattering of disability.

To understand the mattering of disability in accounts of textual recognition requires attention to the materiality of narrative itself. Narratives are produced by intra-acting bodies (throats, tongues, vocal cords, mouths, eyes, hands, in sign language) and material artifacts (paper, pens and pencils, computers, dictation technologies, apps, software programs) within a sea of lived and material encounters and environments. As they emerge, narratives come to move in the world and themselves participate in additional intra-actions as their materiality as printed books, in pdf's, on social media, through sound waves, as visual input, and even through tactile interfaces, is experienced by other intra-acting bodies.[10] But understanding the consequences of the differences emerging in these intra-actions is not always easy to do.

The material encounters involved in producing and experiencing narratives occur amidst waves of dominant and disabled *dis*-attentions that interfere and diffract with one another, producing diffraction patterns. Barad explains that diffraction patterns emerge from "the relative differences (in amplitude and phase) between the overlapping wave components"[11] and that they are important tools for understanding entanglements. "Entanglement"—as Barad uses it—refers to how phenomena are always intra-acting at the same time as apparatuses for perception participate in these intra-actions. The complexity of the dynamics among intra-acting beings, apparatuses, and emergent phenomena makes entanglements exceptionally difficult to study. One approach that quantum physicists have taken is to construct diffraction gratings. A diffraction grating is an apparatus that creates diffraction patterns when waves pass over them; the resulting patterns can be analyzed for what they reveal about the character and behavior of phenomena. Importantly, diffraction patterns can be used to understand the waves being passed through the grating as well as the grating itself. This distinction means that sometimes what we learn is about our own perception and perceptual apparatuses and at other times we learn something about the behavior and practices of phenomena.

As material artifacts that enable attention to entangled phenomena and as processes by which those phenomena emerge, narratives can be understood as diffraction gratings that produce patterns that we can study to understand either what is being passed through the grating (material phenomena and perceptual practices) or the grating itself (narratives as material-discursive artifacts). To work toward the ethical and intentional construction of perceptual apparatuses that enable disability's materialization, we can linger with practices of reading, telling, writing, and analyzing narratives in everyday intra-acting processes. What we learn to pay attention to, and what we anticipate and account for in our stories, are but small fractions of what is actually available for perception. As signs of disability circulate, they create waves of *dis*-attention that diffract and influence disclosures and possibilities for disabling.

In its focus on written narrative, this chapter will recall and return to some of the scenes I have shared in this book of navigating deafness and disability in my academic career. Those experiences, entextualized for this book, are instances where I work to make disability available for readers to notice, not just through my material embodiment as a deaf person but textually within material environments and intra-actions that are always dynamically producing entangled phenomena. This chapter thus extends this book's trajectory to consider the diffraction effects generated among disabled and dominant *dis*-attentions as written texts disperse and move within broader—and often, more mainstream—contexts.

Entextualizing and Dispersing Disability

Dispersal helps us understand how some signs of disability, some forms of *dis*-attention, some disclosures, and some practices of disabling amplify and resonate while others are suppressed or dampened. The material dimensions of texts, including their feel and heft, how they are constructed, and the materials used in that construction, the interfaces and apparatuses that enable their perception, their affective dimensions and relations, and their accessibility—these are all entangled with readers and environments and beings of all kinds. It is in these intra-actions that signs of disability (see introduction) become perceptible as texts disclose (chapter 2) and disable (chapter 3) while dispersing among diffracting waves of dominant and disabled practices of *dis*-attentions (chapter 1). In so doing, these texts and their audiences intra-act to enact agential cuts and place boundaries around phenomena to materialize disability.

While the stories I have told of my own experiences have all moved into various textual forms in order to be part of this book, most were not written prior to their inclusion in this book, and they have morphed and shifted over the publication process. These ongoing changes point to the role that figuring narratives into particular material forms can play in how disability materializes. For instance, in *Sick Building Syndrome*, Michelle Murphy dramatizes an example of this process as she narrates how a new disabling condition came to be identified among office workers in the 1980s. It began, she writes, with individual workers experiencing minor irritations—one rubs an eye, another blows their nose, "a third passes a lozenge to a fourth," until "suddenly a threshold was passed, and now many noticed that they felt unwell." The story continues as "workers, mostly women, staged meetings, collected signatures, filed grievances, conducted informal surveys" in a cycle of repetition among bodies, in different buildings, who, "though many miles apart, . . . heard news of each other through short newspaper articles or TV" until finally, an occupational health problem materialized and "a name circulated, under which all these differences coalesced."[12] This vignette illustrates how the entanglement of interpersonal encounters, textual interfaces (petitions and signatures, grievances, surveys), material environments (1980s office buildings, meeting rooms, floor layouts), and discursive practices all participate in processes of circulation that make disability available for perception.

This materialization involves processes of recontextualization and entextualization as texts move in and out of different contexts. In literacy studies, scholars understand texts not as artifacts or objects but as what Suresh Canagarajah describes as "an activity that is always in the making in its mobility."[13] However, he notes, while written texts are always in motion, they also, to varying degrees, remain relatively stable across contexts. This recursive movement between dynamism and stability, Canagarajah argues, requires that we "hold in tension a decentered text and its artifactual wholeness, its coherence despite its changing and layered nature, its embodiment of meanings despite the constant entextualization of new meanings, and its construction by new social and material contexts despite its ability to change contexts through its 'stabilized for now' status."[14]

The entangled complexity of these tensions is central to textual circulation, which Kate Vieira defines as "the ability of texts to travel, via institutions and people, across space and time,"[15] and it entails taking up the social inequities and power dynamics that always shape—and are shaped by—texts' movements. Too, textual circulation is usefully informed by what Lisa Flores has termed "stoppage" in her historical and cultural analyses of rhetorics surrounding twentieth-century Mexican (im)migration across the US-Mexico border.[16] Stoppage, as Flores forwards it, is a rhetorical mode of racialization in which particular kinds of bodies are classed together in order to control their movement. Just as with bodies, so too with texts and material objects of all kinds. As Vieira puts it, "Race, class, gender, ability, sexuality, language, status, and writers' and publishers' subversive or normative intentions all inform where and how texts move, the hands and institutions through or around which they pass (or don't), and the kinds of meanings that can result."[17]

Both textual mobility and stoppage are useful for understanding the ways that texts and bodies move and intra-act with readers and other material phenomena to shape possibilities for disability to materialize. Texts of all kinds are agential coparticipants in their own emergence and dispersal. They navigate material environments and intra-act with readers' perceptual apparatuses, disclosing and creating waves of different *dis*-attentions that interfere with one another through superpositions and diffraction patterns. When I spent all those hours reading disability memoirs in bed, that choice was motivated by the texts' shape and materiality as physical artifacts that were inviting, comfortable, and familiar to me as printed paperback books. I did not want to read printouts of academic articles or electronic files with my laptop propped on my lap. I did not want to hold a pen or pencil while reading in these specific configurations and times. Through these textual encounters I learned to notice processes of disabling in the texts that came to me, the texts that I stumbled over, the texts that others forwarded to me, the texts that recognized me.

The materiality of authorial bodies also matters for textual production and reception. Despite the focus on texts in the paragraphs above, authorial bodies—the material bodies of writers who compose texts as well as how those bodies are imagined by readers or made available textually—are active participants in texts' production and reception.[18] Stacey Waite helps me understand this tension in *Teaching Queer* as she stresses both the mattering of authorial bodies as well as their frequent elision in various textual encounters. For instance, in noting a general aversion among academics to talking about their bodies, Waite notes that for particular bodies, such attention calling is both unavoidable and oppressive: "Part shame, part fear, part binary of body and mind, this hesitancy can be particularly amplified for queer bodies, or bodies like mine. The queer body always calls attention to what the body knows."[19] Some examples of this bodily knowing that Waite names include the ways that institutions subtly and explicitly invite queer teachers to present themselves as "nice straight folks who will erase themselves as bodies (read: straight people who have invisible bodies unless they are queered in some other way), or who have the luxury of seeming to do so."[20] Lived, material experiences of particular kinds of bodies and their relative perceptibility matters to textual emergence.

Waite also draws on transgender studies' insistence that "identity is inextricably linked to actual material bodies"[21] to argue for the importance of writers' bodies to textual reception. In classrooms, for instance, as Waite points out, teachers always read student writing against a backdrop of encounters with those students—whether sharing space in a physical classroom or interacting online with only a small avatar or videoconference rectangle. This means that for teachers, reading student work necessarily always *also* involves reading students' bodies.[22] As a consequence, readers' perceptions of texts' authors influence how those texts come to mean and circulate. Rebecca Sanchez underscores this point in a discussion of the rise of authorial celebrity as she notes that "public performances trafficked in the audience's desire to read a connection [between personality and text]. The meaning of the works for those who were present became inexorably tied up in their ideas about the body present onstage." As an example, Sanchez takes up a reading performed by Amy Lowell in which audiences reacted negatively to her poem "Spring Day." Sanchez explains listeners' reaction as a reflection of their linking the poet's body with the text of the poem, treating it as "a confessional account of a sensual experience in which they apparently had no desire to fit the noncomformant body of Lowell, who was derided throughout her life for being overweight,"[23] and who was known to be a lesbian. These examples speak to the complex dynamics of stoppage and of practices of textual (im)mobility for understanding dispersal. As Waite puts it, textual encounters are different when one is "reading a book of scholarship by someone whose body you have never seen, whose body you do not know, whose body might intentionally erase itself."[24]

Stoppage and textual (im)mobility each depend on the ways that texts and bodies intra-act and come to be identified as raced, gendered, queered, and disabled. In both Waite's accounting and Sanchez's example, the work of imagination links matter and meaning, a point that Rebecca Dingo amplifies in discussing the role of affect in textual circulation. In her critique of a "Let Girls Learn" video and website purportedly aimed at supporting global girls' empowerment, Dingo explores how some texts gain resonance (or stickiness, following Sara Ahmed) and circulate widely while others slip into relative obscurity. In emphasizing the influence embedded in "residual colonial rhetorics that motivate what audiences presume to already understand and believe about girls in the developing world,"[25] Dingo shows how a video account of Wadley, a fictional Haitian girl, gains widespread circulation across social media while a collection of essays edited by Beverly Bell that depicts real-life Haitian girls' lives and experiences[26] is far less resonant. Examining these accounts and their circulation, Dingo probes whether the texts' different amplification of "typical liberal human rights or neoliberal values" helps explain why one (the fictionalized video playing into myths of empowerment and individual effort) is readily circulated while the other's contrasting representation is largely ignored.[27] To Dingo's attention to affective valences and values, we can add readers' perceptual filtering as audiences encountering the mythical Wadley may find her reinforcing what they already expect while filtering out the contradictory and conflicting details offered by the women telling their stories in Bell's collection. The texts' material features also matter here: Bell's collection was published with a university press and its paperback edition has a $25.95 price point, making it differently accessible as a material artifact to different audiences. Its material existence as a printed book, its cost, the physical and online bookshops and libraries that make the book available, as well as the marketing apparatus surrounding it shape the book's possibilities for circulating physically and electronically and influence how it comes to appear in front of audiences and intra-act with their perceptual apparatuses.

The framework of dispersing that I am forwarding here emphasizes textual materiality, which is shaped by writers' material intra-actions during textual emergence as well as the ways that writers' bodies are recognized and imagined. Textual materiality is also integral to the ways that texts come to readers and the subsequent intra-actions that unfold as readers' perceptual apparatuses enact agential cuts that delineate the boundaries, inclusions, and exclusions around phenomena. In the sections that follow, I first show how authorial intra-actions are consequential for scholarly knowledge production and learning new practices of *dis*-attention. I then take up questions about memoirs written by academics to consider how readers' encounters with texts' material forms matter to the possibilities for disability that emerge.

Knowledge Production and Textual Emergence

Throughout this book, I have told numerous stories that point to moments involved in its making. These everyday experiences of generating academic scholarship work their way into textual emergence in all kinds of ways, and they matter to the knowledge that is produced. Authors may, for instance, make reference to a text's coming-into-being at a particular time (of day, of month, of year, in history, in relation to another time) or place (a writing retreat, home or work office, in stolen moments amidst teaching and other professional commitments), or narrate their lives or their research process, particularly when exceptional circumstances have shaped the work.[28] But such accounts—as frequently as they may occur in academic writing—offer just the scantest traces of the many intra-actions that participate in scholarly publication. As Waite notes, because academics tend to objectify and disembody these processes of knowledge production, such moments are typically hidden or obscured. When these stories and experiences are not surfaced or critically examined, we elide critical elements that shape emergent knowledge as well as possibilities for perception and coming-to-know others. I will briefly take up scholarship in nineteenth- and early-twentieth-century print and material culture for two reasons: first, because emerging textual forms and practices during this period were particularly closely intertwined with changes in bodily perception, interaction, and transformation;[29] and second, because I have spent most of my faculty career in departments populated with leading scholars in this area, which has provided me with readily available opportunities to read and engage my colleagues' work, to attend symposia, lectures, and events, and to learn from serendipitous moments of proximity and connection.

Researchers focused on how nineteenth- and early-twentieth-century Black writers—and Black women writers in particular—navigated material encounters around writing have significantly informed an understanding of the materiality of knowledge production and the intra-actions that support textual circulation. When bodies and texts move together, these intra-actions are consequential for how and what is perceived as well as for knowledge that is produced. Shirley Moody-Turner's work growing a digital archive of Anna Julia Cooper's writing as well as contextualizing and recontextualizing our understanding of Cooper's oeuvre offers a particularly powerful illustration of this point. In "Dear Doctor Du Bois," Moody-Turner draws on letters between Cooper and W. E. B. Du Bois to show how Cooper actively constructed a "collective, dialogical, black publishing praxis" whereby "multiple divergent voices emerge and interact, marginalized black subjectivities find expression, and reductive or dehumanizing discourses are engaged, challenged, and rewritten."[30] This publishing praxis is not just about securing print publication of texts but includes behind-the-scenes editorial interactions in which Cooper lobbies Du Bois as well as criticizes his editorial decisions.[31] And it is not limited only to work that eventually appears in print, as Cooper was not always successful in her efforts to publish her work. Moody-Turner shows these encounters as all significant for Cooper's publishing praxis. Alongside the import she places on Cooper's editorial interactions with Du Bois, Moody-Turner also draws from Cooper's work a recognition of "the importance of interpretive framing in generating productive readings of black women's lives, writings, and histories,"[32] a point she underscores in reviewing the scholarly uptake of Cooper's work in "Prospects for the Study of Anna Julia Cooper." Such efforts emphasize the significance of perceptual apparatuses informed by Black women's lived experience for differently materializing boundaries, properties, and meanings surfacing through texts and publication.[33]

Here, accounts of textual and bodily stoppage as well as mobility profoundly matter to knowledge production, but such accounts—as Moody-Turner's painstaking work shows—can be exceptionally difficult to surface, particularly for writers and knowledge makers whose work has not been widely amplified or circulated. More contemporary scholars have likewise recognized the importance of reviews, citation networks, and scholarly uptake for academic careers. In *Counterstory*, Aja Martinez makes perceptible editorial practices and critical reviews that have limited the citationality, circulation, and reach of work by scholars of color in calling out colleagues and peer reviewers from mainstream journals in rhetoric and writing studies who, she writes, "have told me (sometimes to my face) that my work 'reads like bad fiction,' that it's 'not real research,' and that all I do is write 'biased tales of woe.'"[34] Comments of this sort illustrate how mainstream audiences' resistance to recognizing the relevance and centrality of Martinez's theorizing shaped her book's movement into print.

The scenes of textual emergence that Moody-Turner and Martinez each describe involve a continual interplay between imagined and enacted possibilities, and it is no coincidence that they center on marginalized writers working against mainstream publishing currents. This resistance often requires writers to invent languages and create spaces for their words and ideas to circulate.[35] These acts of imagination and creation emerged over the course of writing; they took place with particular writing tools and materials; and they engaged other actors and material environments that participated in these scenes of textual emergence. In his account of "ethical speculation," forwarded as a theory of desire for writing studies, Jonathan Alexander also centers invention and becoming as he stages a conversation between queer studies and material theories of writing.[36] With ethical speculation, Alexander explicitly names the work of imagination in shaping perception and knowledge. This shaping happens through everyday lived experience as well as in the ways that people account for—that is, story—those experiences, something that José Esteban Muñoz theorizes in his massively influential theory of disidentification, which has been taken up within critical disability studies scholarship.[37] Disidentification, Muñoz notes, describes what happens as queer and negatively racialized people navigate public environments and spaces and repeatedly find themselves butting up against and rubbing alongside "the identity-eroding effects of normativity."[38] Disidentification offers a strategy for subverting this identity erosion by repurposing majoritarian tools and resources to "represent a disempowered politics or positionality that has been rendered unthinkable by the dominant culture."[39] As such, Muñoz's disidentification joins Alexander's "ethical speculation," Moody-Turner's description of Cooper's "collective, dialogical, black publishing praxis," and Martinez's extension of critical race theory counterstory to offer possibilities for ethically reimagining and reshaping perceptions of race and disability alongside experiences of knowledge production.

If *dis*-attending (chapter 1), disclosing (chapter 2), and disabling (chapter 3) are processes whereby lived experiences and perceptual apparatuses are cultivated and shaped through ethical encounters, then they in turn constitute and reconstitute possibilities for what disability can do, be, or know. The insights that Moody-Turner, Martinez, Alexander, and Muñoz offer us stress that how texts and bodies—both imagined and real—circulate and come to intra-act is a crucial element in this process. Here it is important to recall David Valentine's reminder from chapter 1 that "age, race, class, and so on don't merely inflect or intersect with those experiences we call 'gender' and 'sexuality' but rather *shift the very boundaries of what gender and sexuality can mean* in particular contexts."[40] Just as Valentine describes with gender and sexuality, so too with disability: we are not simply "finding" nonnormative bodies but reconstituting the category of disability anew. Given these always-shifting boundaries, this imaginative work can be exceptionally challenging within mainstream contexts that are often overwhelmed or subsumed by dominant *dis*-attentions entangled with myriad other perceptual filters and apparatuses.

Writing disability while engaging in practices of disabling our perceptual apparatuses does not simply involve having a better understanding of how disability takes shape or delineating boundaries around what might and might not be understood as disability. Disabling is not a process of arriving at ever-finer-grained understandings of all the possibilities engendered by signs of disability. Instead, disabling is a process whereby possibilities for and boundaries around disability are made and remade within each intra-action. It thus requires cultivating dis-abled practices of *dis*-attention and recognizing dominant dis-attentions that shape how disclosures come to be perceived. In many mainstream contexts, dominant *dis*-attentions can limit possibilities and subsume complexity and contradiction as ambiguous or deemed-irrelevant or conflicting details get filtered out of perception. As a consequence, mov-ing accounts of writing and texts into (more) widely circulating main-stream contexts and considering different bodies fundamentally changes disability's narrative emergence.[41] The materiality of texts is an active participant in shaping how disability emerges.

To illustrate disability's emergence as scholarly writing moves through various mainstream contexts and different kinds of bodies are called to attention, I take up a series of examples from a subfield of writing stud-ies, writing program administration (WPA), that has been hosting con-versations about the relationships between academics' bodies and their scholarly and professional work. I begin with Amy Vidali's "Disabling Writing Program Administration," in which she narrates her experience with depression against a backdrop of embodied accounts of WPA work. "Disabling" was published as a print academic journal article available to journal subscribers (members of the Council of Writing Program Administrators) as well as a pdf available to subscribers through the journal's archives and through academic libraries. The affordances of an academic journal's textual forms and its print and digital materiality par-ticipate in making Vidali's body—and WPA bodies in general—available for noticing. In "Disabling," Vidali describes the frequency with which WPAs narrate experiences of overwork, stress, and exhaustion that have disabling effects, some of which require them to give up WPA work or leave academia. These accounts do not point to a wide range of disability experiences as they focus largely on anxiety and depression seemingly caused by the conditions of WPA work and potentially cured or allevi-ated once people stop being WPAs. Vidali notes that this orientation to disability elides possibilities for other materializations: that WPAs may be disabled before they take on their roles; that not all disability experi-ences can be cured or alleviated; and that WPAs have disabilities other than anxiety and depression.[42]

To resist these dominant *dis*-attentions, Vidali shares her own expe-riences with anxiety and depression—disabilities that are not helped by a highly demanding and stressful position, but that were not caused by her WPA role. Throughout the essay Vidali uses narratives to teach readers how to *dis*-attend differently. Short vignettes are interspersed throughout the text and formally distinguished from the main text by being indented and italicized. Her first vignette describes a meeting with her chair where she gets a lower-than-expected annual evaluation. In response, she starts crying and (presumably to avoid her chair) begins "going in to the department office on weekends" to do her photocopying.[43] Vidali acknowledges that many WPAs will recognize this experience as just "a typical tale of WPA work," but goes on to note that this reaction is shaped by dominant *dis*-attentions that direct focus away from disability: "In my mini-narrative above, I have emphasized my stress and hard work, as WPA narratives often do, but have elided the depression that informed but was only tangentially caused by my WPA work. Put another way, when I read this narrative, I know it's a story of depression, but WPAs may read it as a typical tale of WPA work."[44]

Vidali's vignette shows crying as the work of the body, as well as photocopying, while both disappear in WPA work and in the writing that accompanies it. Too, the ease with which many WPAs may dismiss this mini-narrative as simply "a story of WPA work" resonates with the dominant *dis*-attentions that led Tonia's colleagues (chapter 3) to materialize anything-but-disability in their everyday workplace interactions. In these ways, mainstream contexts actively participate in amplifying some perceptions and interpretations of particular sensory input while resisting or dampening other possibilities.

As the essay unspools, Vidali increasingly disables her vignettes. By the end of the article, her vignettes offer up imaginative possibilities for narrating disability and WPA work that resist dominant *dis*-attentions that might seek to redeem her depression into a celebratory account. Vidali's immersion in the field of disability studies put her in company with many other disabled scholars, and her own experiences of navigating disability disclosures in her life as well as in her scholarship[45] have led to connection and community among others who understand and identify with those experiences. Her proximity to tenure at the time of writing this essay and her previous scholarly productivity influenced her experience of moving this piece through publication and navigating reviewer and editorial feedback.[46] Vidali's insights about and careful readings of

WPAs' bodies has been integral to my own thinking in this project as I have worked to understand how signs of disability take shape. But when we ask what is included and excluded as perceptual apparatuses enact agential cuts that draw boundaries around phenomena, we must return again to questions of WPA bodies and their mattering and how that mattering is made available for perception in these narratives.[47]

When experiences of disability are entangled with other forms of systemic oppression and institutional racism, the boundaries around disability take on very different shapes and forms (see also Tonia's account in chapter 3). For many Black and minoritized bodies, identifying with disability brings very different risks and consequences than it does for white bodies. The accounts of overwork, anxiety, depression, and stress that Vidali analyzes generally do not take up the mattering of the authors' racialized bodies, potentially reinforcing a long-standing critique that much disability studies work focuses on white disabled people to the exclusion of other possibilities for disability's materialization. Indeed, in a 2016 symposium on "Challenging Whiteness and/in Writing Program Administration and Writing Programs," Sherri Craig calls out the paucity of stories in the field from people of color, arguing that this absence, "whether intentional or not, silently and systematically reaffirms the marginality of non-white, unprivileged narratives."[48] The few stories that have been published, Craig notes, tell of "exclusion and physical and emotional displacement," leading her to wonder, "Is that it? Is this the only narrative the journal has for people of color? Why this?" The limited overt recognition of the texture of racialized mattering leads to a narrow conceptualization of these experiences. As Craig wonders, she experiences emotional ups and downs that she connects to the stages of grief, including "depression about my position as a person of color in WPA studies."[49] While Craig uses depression in a colloquial rather than clinical sense here, when considered alongside stories told by other Black WPAs,[50] her reference nevertheless suggests the need—as Therí Pickens urges with Blackness and madness—to read in and between the text's folds to understand how disability might materialize in Black WPA narratives. Such a reading requires a perceptual apparatus informed by attention to race's mattering in everyday lived experience as well as grounding in scholarly approaches that center Black disabled onto-epistemologies, such as Pickens's *Black Madness :: Mad Blackness*,

Moya Bailey and Izetta Mobley's "Black feminist disability framework," and Sami Schalk and Jina B. Kim's "feminist-of-color disability studies."[51]

A reading and perceptual apparatus informed by this body of scholarship might begin with the tropes of overwork and stress that Vidali recognizes in WPA narratives and that Jina B. Kim and Alexis Pauline Gumbs each acknowledge in women-of-color feminist academics' experiences.[52] The physical and mental consequences of long-term conditions of overwork and stress have come to be recognized as features of academic life more generally and not just WPA work, given the increasing neoliberalization of higher education (see also chapter 3). These conditions for academic labor, including cultures of hyperproductivity, have been critiqued by disability studies scholars such as Akemi Nishida for the ways that they amplify dominant practices of *dis*-attention to embodied mattering and have debilitating effects on bodies and minds.[53] These effects are compounded at the intersections of race and disability. Bailey and Mobley note, for instance, that because of the ways that Black bodies have been valued for their labor and productivity, "the stakes for identifying as disabled, or acknowledging a compromised relationship to labor and the ability to generate capital, is often not a viable option for most Black people."[54] Bailey puts this in more personal terms in a blog post for the *Sociological Review*: "As a Black queer chronically ill woman, I work extra hard and produce in excess in the hopes of thwarting a latent imposter syndrome and my internalized ableist standards. My overworking and overproduction prove necessary in a misogynoirist academic culture; however, the physical toll on my body and others like mine is palpable."[55] These insights, considered among a broader terrain of embodied mattering and how it is made available for noticing in personal encounters and academic scholarship, require us to ask after the mattering of race as it becomes available on WPA bodies and the diffraction patterns that are caused by these different waves of *dis*-attention.

Ethical practices of disabling require conscious attention across experiences that matter to how we materialize disability. If disability is imagined predominantly as white and female, for instance, what is filtered out of noticing, assumed to be irrelevant, or actively erased? If "trauma, violence, and pain"[56] are so much part of Black women's everyday experience that they recede into the background, how can that instead be foregrounded, made available for noticing, and thus support conditions for change? Disabling our perceptual apparatuses calls not just for individual academics learning to productively *dis*-attend (although I am advocating for this) but for entire systems of knowledge production to be reconstituted.[57] Learning from our "bodies of knowledge," as Waite urges us to do, and as the contributors to Perryman-Clark and Craig's *Black Perspectives in Writing Program Administration* enact, requires critical attention to what is filtering through—and out of—our perceptual apparatuses as well as being made available, or not available, in the stories we tell. These stories emerge from the everyday encounters and practices that shape our academic lives and come to circulate within our professional discourses. White academics' elision of race is not a testament to the lack of mattering of race, and addressing systemic inequities requires that they (myself included) recognize the palpable presence of whiteness as well as its investment in filtering attention to race from many white people's perceptual apparatuses. In this way, the dominant *dis*-attentions that filter or background perceptions of race in materializing disability matter to how texts—academic articles and otherwise—circulate.

Texts' material forms participate in these perceptual apparatuses, a point that the open-access 2021 special issue of *WPA: Writing Program Administration* makes apparent. This issue's table of contents featured article titles and author names but added a brief italicized description of the authors.[58] These descriptions, much like other not-generally-common practices in academic journals such as including author photos, point to ways that textual forms and infrastructures beyond article content also participate in making available various means of perceiving authorial bodies. It is worth further exploring how some of these textual infrastructures are differently available depending on how the journal circulates. For instance, the front matter of the journal is generally only available to those who access the full issue, whether by downloading an open-access pdf for those issues made available in this way, by receiving a print copy as a journal subscriber, or by accessing a bound copy of the journal in a library. Most academic databases—such as Gale Academic OneFile, the database I use at my current institution to navigate this journal's archives—only provide access to individual articles, not the journal's front matter or other paratextual elements of the print journal. And, as the discussion above of authors' experiences with editorial practices and processes of peer review further reinforces, these editorial practices and processes are likewise intra-acting participants in textual circulation.

The scholarship I have engaged in this chapter points to relationships between textures of lived experience, textual materiality, and textual circulation for how disability comes to be noticed and is made available for noticing. Accounting for racialized perceptions and experience is thus an essential element of boundary making around disability. Our perceptual apparatuses are built through lived experience and honed and developed through intra-actions with materials, bodies, and environments that are all part of bringing written texts into existence. The preceding discussion centered on how narrative choices made amidst scholarly publication processes—which are always material, involving academics' bodies, as well as those of editors and audiences—participate in disability's emergence as a phenomenon. The next section takes these questions about disability perceptibility and processes of disabling within mainstream contexts to consider the burgeoning genre of disability memoir and life writing. While my discussion of academic scholarship centered on conditions for knowledge generation and academics' bodily mattering for textual circulation, my discussion of disability memoir will center on readers' materiality/embodiment and the intra-actions they participate in with texts in various material forms.

Producing Disability Memoirs

At the start of this chapter, I narrated my early engagement with (white-dominated) disability studies scholarship as one facilitated by reading memoirs before bed. In the ten years since that sabbatical, my interest in disability memoir and life writing has not waned. My desire for disabled stories and the affective pleasures of reading about people's lives are a large part of this motivation, but my interest is also material, and involves my own and others' disabled and racialized embodiments. For instance, I love the tactile and sensory experience of wandering among stacks of books and rows of bookshelves in stores and libraries. I often drag my fingers along the books' spines, feeling my fingers bump up and down against the different textures. I take in the visual arrangement of books and read the categories displayed on shelves organizing the books. I love the musty old-book smell deep in libraries' stacks and the mingling of smells of coffee and new paper in many contemporary bookstores. However, these experiences and my affective relations to them are also artifacts of my whiteness and physical mobility: many people navigate these experiences differently, whether because of geographic or physical inaccessibility or because libraries and businesses are closed to them. Such experiences might be about elevators' access to certain floors, the ability to reach or carry heavy books, or where they are stored, such as in special collections or other accessible-only-by-permission spaces. Too, questions about who has access to libraries or the neighborhoods where they are located, and who can move freely in them all point to policies and practices that restrict what kinds of bodies can comfortably move in the ways I have just described.

In her book on the explosion of memoir and life writing, Julie Rak shows these material encounters as integral to the popularity of memoir as a genre. While they are not a central focus of scholarship outside of book history, Rak argues that "the material circumstances of book acquisition" are essential to an understanding of how texts come to circulate and are encountered by readers. To illustrate this point, Rak analyzes the physical elements and spatial arrangements of a set of chain and independent bookstores in Canada and argues for a material account of genre classification, in which she shows genres emerging from a complex entanglement of elements, including book arrangements, shelves and store furniture, employees' job descriptions, store cultures, labels and categories organizing books, and broader practices of book classification (e.g., the Dewey Decimal System's division between fiction and nonfiction).[59] Black librarian Dorothy Porter's work offers particular insight on the materiality of classification systems and how they make phenomena available for perception. In explaining how Porter worked "to dismantle the tools she learned in library school and remake them to capaciously delineate blackness,"[60] Laura Helton argues that Porter's efforts show "how the tools that beget access to reading objects also organize the imperatives and imaginaries that beget reading subjects."[61] In these relationships between access and audience, Porter's work picks up the thread of imagination that loops through this chapter, emphasizing how imaginative acts can themselves materialize phenomena.

Significantly, however, these acts can also function to elide and erase: "Porter was also a careful observer of how categorization could hide a text—another way to deny access even when the doors of a library were open."[62] That the acts of arranging, classifying, and organizing information enacted through Porter's librarianship were deeply material and "performed by women who produced lists and card files, and not rhetoric or verse"[63] is yet another reminder of the materiality of knowledge production that is central to disability's emergence.

Just as Porter critiqued and revised logics for organizing and finding Blackness in libraries and information infrastructures, materializing disability in existing bookstore and library classification systems remains challenging. For as long as I have been writing and thinking about disability memoir and accounts of disabled lives, I have been navigating bookstores' and libraries' material infrastructures and environments, working to make disability available for noticing within my perceptual apparatus. Few libraries or bookstores have a section labeled "disability memoir," so I have learned to look for other cues. Sometimes there is a general memoir category. Within this category, I always need to do additional work to determine a memoir's relationship to disability, making some inferences based on the book's title, its marketing description, or the images on its cover. At other times memoirs that I might incorporate into a disability category are tucked in bookstore sections titled "health and wellness" or "sociology" or "psychology" or "social sciences." When I lived in Delaware, my local public library had a large section packed with memoirs that showcased many older books than would generally be available for sale in a bookstore that prioritizes new and recently published texts. University libraries, which use the Library of Congress classification system, categorize these texts either within a specific subsection on disability or under medical categories.[64] Here again, the logics and materials of classification shape what is findable and how.[65] Searching for disability memoir online feels even more challenging than in the in-person searching I often do in libraries and bookstores. Search interfaces and algorithms do not resonate with my own perceptual apparatus—in fact, they often seem at odds with it—and the sorts of things I am interested in are not always the things that come up when I am searching. While "consumers also bought" recommendations sometimes return useful suggestions, I mostly find online searching frustrating at least in part because I am limited in what I can experience of the book's materiality: I can't pick it up, make inferences based on its weight, the paper it uses, the font size and appearance, and more. I also do not have full understanding of how the online algorithms—which are themselves biased in ways that have inequitable outcomes on search results—have brought any particular book to the top of a search result.[66]

These examples point to ways that librarians, researchers, knowledge producers, and readers all participate in material processes of circulating disability. No matter where I am, finding disabled (not just disability-related) memoirs feels like a sophisticated guessing game during which I put to work the perceptual apparatus that I have been building through my immersion in disability studies, a life lived as a deaf woman, and my enjoyment of reading lots of different kinds of things. Within mainstream publishing contexts, the challenges around making phenomena perceptible are particularly acute for those whose experiences do not fit into readily available narrative plot lines. This point has been repeatedly acknowledged in disability studies since the late 1990s when G. Thomas Couser pointed to the prevalence of cancer memoirs that end by narrating the author's recovery as well as the dearth of narratives that conclude with the author's death.[67] In addition to the fact that people with terminal cancer may not have time and/or energy to give to writing, it is also the case that memoirs that end in death, or that refuse to conclude with a "happily ever after" run the risk of, well, not being very popular. Publishers' increasing reliance on predictions about popularity have led to a more risk-averse publishing environment and greater homogenization in mainstream publishing. A *New York Times* feature on Madeline McIntosh, the CEO of Penguin Random House, links this phenomenon to the algorithms that drive online shopping. Because the algorithms look for the books that are already selling well, those books are what shoppers encounter when searching online. This situation, paired with the fact that publishers have relatively little control over what readers come across as they shop online (in contrast to the ways publishers can influence the material experience of shopping at a physical bookstore)[68] results in "an algorithmic marketplace that serves up mostly the hits, driving a cycle so self-fulfilling it's nearly tautological: Best sellers sell the best because they are best sellers."[69] This emphasis then pressures writers to produce work that will satisfy assumptions about market demand and what will sell.[70] These calculations take on other shapes and emphasis at different publishing houses given the ways that publishers imagine their reading audience in broad or narrow terms.

It remains exceptionally challenging to move disabled perspectives into mainstream spheres, to resist the mainstream waves of *dis*-attention that not only erase disabled people's perceptions of the world but, when they do point to disability, often emphasize accounts of white disabled people overcoming their disabilities.[71] Here, dominant and disabled *dis*-attentions, storytellers' perceptual apparatuses, textual materiality, and circulation networks all intra-act with readers' perceptual apparatuses to materialize (particular phenomena of) disability. It is not all that surprising to me that the memoirs I come across when browsing bookstores, whether in person or online, are hit-or-miss where it comes to disability and disabling. Yet, even as I do not know for sure what I am going to find when I open the kinds of mass-published books that are most often for sale in bookstores, available on library shelves, or at the top of my Internet searches, what pulls me to open the book in the first place is some sort of sign of disability, something that grabs my attention and suggests to me that this book might, when intra-acting with me as a reader and my perceptual apparatus and my practices of *dis*-attention, materialize disability in some way. This searching is highly inefficient. There are so many memoirs, and disability is in almost all of them in some way, shape, or form. I can't read anything without noticing a sign of disability somewhere. There are the (ghostwritten) celebrity memoirs most often by famous white disabled people, almost always illustrated with the celebrity author's face on the cover. I sometimes struggle to read these all the way through. I am not really all that interested in the celebrity memoir, or even many of the accounts of disability and non-normative embodiment published by mass-market publishers, prominently displayed on the shelves at a bookstore, or at the top of online search algorithms. Again and again, these texts emphasize problematic tropes of overcoming or tread familiar plot lines in showing disability to a mainstream, imagined-as-nondisabled audience. I find that I have the most success with texts recommended by other disability studies scholars and disability activists.

My interest in diffracting waves of *dis*-attention also pushes me to consider books that do not obviously display signs of disability. I pull all kinds of books off shelves trying to learn more about how academics write their bodies into their texts. I start collecting faculty memoirs and essay collections that feature narratives of faculty life. The list grows on a near-daily basis. Some are mass-market books from writers who are (or were, at the time the books were published) faculty members, such as Roxane Gay's *Hunger* and Kiese Laymon's *Heavy*. Others are published through academic presses (Christina Crosby's *A Body, Undone*, Anand Prahlad's *Secret Life of a Black Aspie*, Cheryl Savageau's *Out of the Crazywoods*), small independent presses (Elaine Richardson's *From PHD to PhD*), or even self-published (Ann Millett-Galant's *Re-Membering*).[72] As I read these memoirs, I hope to learn how these accounts of embodied experience might connect with disability while at the same time working to notice how *dis*-attentions shaped by my lived experiences of whiteness and deafness are filtering these accounts. Here the limits of my perceptual apparatus matter for the inclusions and exclusions I am enacting as I learn new disabled ways of *dis*-attending and materializing disability.

To illustrate this process, I will take up the example of Porochista Khakpour's *Sick: A Memoir*, which was published as a trade book by Harper Perennial in 2018.[73] I first came across the book when it was praised on a disability studies listserv I am part of. Where and how did disability materialize beginning with my first encounters with the book? An important sign is its recommendation on the listserv, which is what motivates me to add it to the growing pile of memoirs in my office. There is also its title, which evokes a medical orientation and the management of health that is a focal point of the book. Once I am touching the book, other signs emerge. I examine the images on the front cover while running my hand over its smooth texture and flip it over to check out the back. My edition has two images on the front cover: a black and white photo of Khakpour showing her in bed wearing a nasal cannula and with dark hair spilling around her face on a pillow. Below the photograph, there is a colorful image of yellow, pink, white, and blue pills scattered together. In an interview with the *LA Times*, Khakpour explained that the cover photo was a selfie that she took "back in 2011 or 2012 when I'd just be in bed for hours at a time either in hospitals or at my doctor's office, taking photos, like, Who am I? What happened to me? How do I feel right now? How am I managing?"[74] This front cover image dramatically contrasts with the author photo on the final pages of the book, which shows her wearing a stylish leather jacket and large cats-eye-shaped glasses while posing with her right hand on her hip.

My copy is a mass-market paperback. Its paper is slightly rough, is highly flexible, and rips easily. I can tell it will not have long-term durability, a prediction that has been borne out given how beat up it now looks after my reading and rereading of it while writing this book. The cheaper paper, as compared with the archival-weight paper used in many of the other memoirs in my collection,[75] makes *Sick* less expensive, lighter, easier to circulate, easier to assign in undergraduate and graduate classes, easier to get in bookstores.[76] I read the acknowledgments and riffle the pages, visually apprehending elements of the typesetting, the spacing between lines, numerous features of the book that tell me something about what to expect. Before I have even begun to engage with Khakpour's prose, I am processing the book's materiality as I am able to navigate it.

Other readers will materialize different phenomena from the book's materiality, a point that is especially evident when one considers the different formats through which readers can encounter the book. Readers might download the e-book to a tablet or a proprietary e-reader using a variety of apps and book-selling platforms. They might listen to it through a screen reader or as a professionally narrated audiobook. They might navigate a computer or web-based interface. These will all make available different features of the book—so my account of how I personally handle physical books and the meanings I make from them is simultaneously collective and idiosyncratic, as Friedman and Zerubavel explain about perception generally (see chapter 1). As Georgina Kleege, who is blind, explains, "There's listening, and then there's *listening*"; in the latter mode, she prefers to listen to texts read by a synthesized voice "at a rate of about 400 words a minute" and perceives the text in particular ways in her practice of listening as "an active pursuit, an attentive selection and absorption of meaningful sounds."[77] Kleege's account resonates with the sociological framework of perception Friedman and Zerubavel help us understand, and shows its imbrication with embodied materiality and intra-actions with a material surround.

Part of the materiality of Khakpour's book that I intra-act with is its marketing apparatus—which will be differently available to different readers depending on book modality, material surround, readers' embodiment, and perceptual apparatus. There are multiple blurbs on the front and back covers and more printed on the first few pages inside the front cover. The blurb featured prominently at the top of the front cover praises Khakpour's "struggle toward health" as well as her intelligence and intimacy. But I am a little disappointed after I finish reading all the blurbs. There is one highlighted on the back cover that reads, "This book gives a voice—a fierce, booming, brutally honest voice—to the millions of people silently suffering with invisible illnesses of their own." I recognize in this blurb the familiar trope of voicelessness, of living with disability as a life of suffering. I am perhaps too familiar with dominant *dis*-attentions that filter perceptions of chronic illness to reveal it as pain and suffering and *only* pain and suffering, eliding other possibilities. This blurb further reminds me that while my own perceptual apparatus is highly attuned to experiences of chronic illness as well as racialized, gendered, and economically stratified health disparities[78] as connected to disability's materialization, for many others, disability will be kept at a distance and possibly not materialize at all.

I become intensely interested in the question of whether Khakpour herself is aware of disability as a cultural (and not just medical) category as she writes; I wonder how she seeks to materialize disability within her account. In this, I am conscious of my own *dis*-attentions, built from a life lived as a white woman with a relatively predictable and generally readily recognized physical disability and want to avoid imposing them on the experiences Khakpour narrates. My interaction with the text as a particular kind of reader and with a particular apparatus for perceiving signs of disability is deeply consequential for the phenomena that ultimately materialize. I have not come to this book in a vacuum, after all: it has been recommended by other people who, I know, are also looking for disability everywhere they turn. In the entry for *Sick* in a massive two-volume encyclopedia of disability life writing, Coleman Nye reads Khakpour as resisting notions of cure and as showing her experience with Lyme disease as "inextricably linked to other aspects of bodily unease,"[79] as well as to the sociomaterial environment in which she experiences it. But the narrative resistance that scholars like Nye might identify or that emerges in some of Khakpour's interviews is ignored entirely in most of the book's paratext.[80] For instance, of the ten paragraph-length blurbs printed on (or inside) my copy of the book, none uses the word "disability" to describe Khakpour's experience or the story she recounts of living with late-stage Lyme disease, although words like "health," "vibrant," "strong," and "wellness" appear alongside "illness," "sickness," "vulnerable," "disease," "physical suffering," "addiction," "infection," and "bodily and emotional needs." Two blurbs present *Sick* in victorious terms: "Miraculously, *Sick* emerges as a force of life" and "*Sick* is a triumph of the imagination as she holds her heart out to you." The blurbs again and again return to the language of celebration, setting off waves of *dis*-attention that feel to me like efforts to materialize not-disability and redeem the badness and pain of illness and vulnerability.

Now, the book's marketing apparatus is not the most important means by which disability might materialize: I am more interested in Khakpour's writing than the blurbs. I also realize that authors do not have control over their blurbs or book covers. But this marketing is also important for me to pay attention to for the ways that it repeatedly reinforces dominant forms of *dis*-attention and teaches me something about how this text will or might circulate. Orientations to disability that are largely shaped by ableist perspectives come to be readily amplified in ways that can subsume *dis*-attentions taught, learned, and performed by disabled people themselves. The diffraction patterns that emerge as my perceptual apparatus filters my perceptions of *Sick* are influenced by waves of *dis*-attention that emphasize disability as deficit or loss and that persistently link authority around disability to doctors and medical professionals rather than disabled people themselves.

Complex relations among systems of power and oppression thus shape the different waves of *dis*-attention that simultaneously materialize disability in particular ways and obscure other possibilities for its materialization. For instance, against the celebrations of Khakpour's prose in the blurbs, I am noticing the potential for other *dis*-attentions, such as those informed by what Schalk and Kim describe as "the logics of gender and sexual regulation that undergird racialized resource deprivation,"[81] including around access to and treatment within health care contexts, to shape disability's emergence here. As these diffracting *dis*-attentions move through my perceptual apparatus, they enact a set of superpositions that matter to how I engage with Khakpour's words. Because I have been bombarded with these ableist ideas about disability,

I am paying extra-careful attention to Khakpour's words, working to understand what she is communicating. The first words from Khakpour (potentially) sit just opposite the copyright page in the form of a medical disclaimer: "This book contains my personal story. I am not a medical professional, and therefore, the inadvertent advice and information I share throughout this book is in no way intended to be construed as medical advice. If you know or suspect that you have a health problem, it is recommended that you seek the advice of your physician or other professional advisor before embarking on any medical program or treatment."[82]

I pause on this page and read and reread this disclaimer. I do not know if Khakpour herself wrote those words or if they were suggested to her by lawyers concerned about legal liability, but the use of first person and the emphasis on "my personal story" associate the words with Khakpour's authorial voice. "Inadvertent advice and information" is a striking phrase: inadvertent, with its meaning of unintended or unplanned, when paired with "advice and information," marks a difference from "medical advice." In *Sick*, readers will learn about Khakpour's experience with chronic (also known as late-stage) Lyme disease, which is a contested illness and has scant medical consensus about treatment. This lack of consensus means that some readers may come to her book seeking to learn more about her treatment, perhaps to get ideas about what might work for them too. However, as this note makes clear, Khakpour's experience is not medical advice, and if you, the reader, "know or suspect that you have a health problem, it is recommended" (by whom?) that you should get other advice from medical professionals. This odd paragraph imagines several potential audiences for the book, from people who know nothing about Lyme to people who have experienced chronic Lyme and searched everywhere for help. The legalistic and distanced tone of the third sentence, which begins with, "If you know or suspect that you have a health problem," evokes for me a monotone commercial disclaimer for a prescription medication and contrasts with the intimacy of the preceding sentences. I wonder what went into crafting this disclaimer. I wonder how much Khakpour pushed back, what kind of interactions led to this statement. This note offers hints of legal wrangling around language as texts go through publication processes—a wrangling that enacts material consequences on texts and that can, for readers and authors alike, have violent effects through the persistence of particular names and terminology, for instance.[83] It reminds me that texts and words matter, that they do things in the world and have consequences. It refuses the illusion that this is simply one person's story, disembodied and separate from innumerable intra-acting encounters leading to this book's publication.

After a dedication, epigraphs, and a title page, the book proper begins with a two-and-a-half page "Author's Note" in which Khakpour lays out as best she can the few facts she knows about Lyme disease. The Author's Note functions in some similar ways to Vidali's effort in "Disabling WPA" to teach her readers how to notice signs of disability in her vignettes. Khakpour opens with, "It seems impossible to tell this story without getting the few certainties out of the way, the closest one can come to 'facts.'"[84] After noting how difficult it is to define Lyme ("to pinpoint this disease, to define it, in and of itself is something of a labor"), she shares a series of scientific facts and figures, naming the bacteria that causes Lyme (*Borrelia burdorferi*), offering an estimate of the money she has spent on Lyme treatments, describing disease stages, and sharing research data on the costs of Lyme disease in the United States.[85]

This Author's Note ripples with *dis*-attention. One wave involves what Jay Dolmage describes in *Disability Rhetoric* as a set of disability myths that circulate various kinds of meanings for disability. For Dolmage, each myth "is a *misplacement* of meaning," acting as stereotypes and tropes that rhetorically "provide material for a wide range of expressions, whether through compressed analogies or longer narratives."[86] The first in his list is "Disability as Pathology," which he describes by explaining that "there is almost always a moment in a narrative in which the disabled character is 'explained' by a doctor or nurse, who provides a sort of WebMD overview of their pathology. Disability rarely circulates in popular culture without a medicalized explanation and definition."[87] And it is here that I notice another wave of *dis*-attention moving through the Author's Note as Khakpour works to disclose disability. While we can read Khakpour as giving in to popular demands for "explanation," she does so after opening with, "It seems impossible to tell this story without getting the few certainties out of the way."[88] Why is it impossible? What necessitates this act of "getting the few certainties out of the way"? These facts are referenced throughout the memoir, not by being quoted but by providing foundational elements for a perceptual apparatus that, once made available to readers, might enable them to *dis*-attend differently. In this Author's Note, then, Khakpour frontloads as many signs of disability as she can in order to provide a context for reading her book. The "certainties" reinforce Khakpour's own expertise, which constitutes a third, disabled *dis*-attention diffracting the text. While her disclaimer explicitly asserts that she is "not a medical professional," the Author's Note nevertheless lays out the depth and range of her expertise on Lyme disease. This extra-narrative positioning then enables her readers to recognize and take up some of the signs of disability and disclosures enacted by the text once she begins telling her account. The story she tells throughout *Sick* is one of living with disability and chronic illness as an immigrant and as a woman of color, but it is not a medicalized account. She does not tell the story of how her diagnosis defines her, or how medicalized frames position and situate her. Instead, the memoir disables as it works to teach readers new ways to *dis*-attend, to understand and notice what it means to be sick, and it does so by offering content that resists the book's material architecture and paratext.

The Author's Note is immediately followed by a vignette titled "On the Wrong Body" that offers a two-page description of Khakpour's body—a means, alongside the photographs on the cover and at the very back of the book—of making available her physical appearance and various forms of embodied presence and their relationship to the portrait of chronic Lyme she offers in the book. It is here that she writes, "At some point, with chronic illness and disability, I grew to feel at home. My body was wrong, and through data, we could prove that." This is the first use of the word "disability" in the text, and it comes early enough to contrast with the elisions of and euphemisms for disability in the blurbs and marketing copy.

The interactions Khakpour describes throughout the book contrast with the knowledge—such as it is, of a condition as contested as late-stage Lyme—that she reveals in her Author's Note. She is an expert, she has significant rhetorical skill, and yet she is frequently surrounded by people who think she is not—people who deny and dismiss her lived experience. These are also often people who have some control over her access to treatment or whom Khakpour is relying on for help. This framing contextualizes how Khakpour early in the book narrates her experience of a car accident and its aftermath. When she finally goes to the hospital after the accident, her editor (who accompanied her to the hospital) has to remind her that she is there not for complications of her Lyme disease but to get checked out post-accident. As Khakpour puts it, "I had been to the hospital so many times for my Lyme disease, not just explaining but overexplaining, as if I had something to hide. Lyme is a disease that many in the medical profession, unless they specialize in it, find too controversial, too full of unknowns, to fully buy it as legitimate."[89] And sure enough, when she needs to ask for an MRI instead of a CT scan, she has to reveal her diagnosis of Lyme. When she refuses the CT scan, the ER doctor sends her away with a prescription for Tylenol. In this scene, Khakpour reveals to her readers a kind of medical entitlement to narrative, in which medical professionals compel disclosures of various kinds only to refuse patient authority.[90] These experiences shape her—not just in providing material for the book but in creating the book and the conditions of possibility for narrative. These experiences, in other words, are part of what necessitates the Author's Note that is our first real encounter with Khakpour's prose and style in the book.

As I engage with Khakpour's words, I recognize her text as part of a tradition of disability memoirs that disable—texts that invoke and address disabled audiences and resist dominant forces of *dis*-attention. They do so by helping their readers build perceptual apparatuses for materializing disability and by offering possibilities for enabling and resisting forces of *dis*-attention in varying degrees. Like many writers who use language to transport experiences across time and space, Khakpour works to make disability available for them as readers. But she is also navigating environments where her experiences are shaped by readers, both those who materially interact with her in the publication process and also those imagined/potential readers enacted by the press and shaped by dominant *dis*-attentions that make the book accessible to them through particular marketing frames and apparatuses. In the book's epilogue, Khakpour highlights once again the material interactions leading to the shape of the book that ultimately got published. She writes, "And then this book, The Book I Sold. The Book I Sold was a story of triumph, of how a woman dove into the depths of addiction and illness and got well. She got herself better. She made it. The Book I Sold might even imply you can do it too. Or anyone can. Who knows. The Book I Sold was never written past a bare-bones proposal."[91]

Listeners familiar with disability studies will immediately recognize in "The Book I Sold" the common tropes of disability narrative, of the return to wellness, what Dolmage has called the "Kill or Cure" disability myth in which any representation of a disabled person needs to end with them either dying or being cured. In an interview, Khakpour commented on "The Book I Sold," saying, "I mean, what a fake book that would have been," going on to elaborate: "The Book I Sold would have been a pretty crappy book. I mean, I wish I was better, and I wish I wasn't going through all this, but I don't think that book would have been a good book, because it would have just been: Ta dah!"[92]

Khakpour's comment here is a reminder that disability does not materialize out of nothing. It is a deeply material imbrication with the world that becomes available for perception through story. She also raises questions about the kinds of stories it is possible to tell about disability, stressing just how hard it can be to tell a story about disability that does not end on a happy note, exactly the kind of happy note Khakpour points to with "The Book I Sold." In this way, "The Book I Sold" suggests one way that Khakpour's experience of writing this book changed—disabled—her.

The challenges of making disability available for perception within written texts points to the work that goes into bringing them into existence. Writers of all kinds negotiate a sea of encounters that all, in different ways, consequentially shape texts' final appearance and circulation. Lived experiences with disability and practices of learning to *dis*-attend differently matter as well. Readers coparticipate with texts as material artifacts to shape how they appear and circulate. Understanding how disability comes to be perceived and materialize as texts circulate within dynamic material environments, then, is to consider complexly entangled intra-actions, infused with desire and imagination, and constituted through material beings and perceptual apparatuses.

Epilogue

Disorientations

In the preceding chapters of this book, I have forwarded a framework of signs of disability that coalesces around four conceptual terms—"*dis*-attending," "disclosing," "disabling," and "dispersing"—that can help us learn to attend to the signs of disability all around us. This framework has emerged through a methodology and data set centered on stories and storying that reveal signs of disability as dynamic, engaged, and lived practices in all kinds of everyday scenes. But signs of disability, as this book has tried to show, are also highly disorienting. *Dis*-attention is, as I note in chapter 1, a purposefully polyvalent neologism intended to trip us up, slow us down, and twist us around as we try to learn what it means to notice a world made up of and with disability. As the material world becomes sensory input that intra-acts with our perceptual apparatuses, dominant practices of *dis*-attention work to make disability available for noticing only in highly constrained or narrowly authorized ways, and often act in the service of coopting or sanitizing disability.

To resist such ways of perceiving disability requires us to learn to attend differently to the world's disclosures. It requires us to do the hard work of intentionally reshaping our perceptual apparatuses. One way to move, then, is to learn from perceptual apparatuses shaped by experiences of disability amidst complex lives and environments. It also means disabling—in the sense I suggest for this word in chapter 3—practices of *dis*-attention by building and sustaining meaningful relationships and entanglements among disabled onto-epistemologies. The final core term of this book, "dispersing," takes up questions of how disability is made available for noticing as texts take shape and move. Writers' bodies matter in many different ways to how a text materializes into being, and intra-actions of all kinds over the course of composing participate in texts' emergence as well as in the ways that a text comes to circulate. As texts come to readers, their materiality intra-acts with readers' perceptual apparatuses to shape possibilities for disability and its coming into being.

In this epilogue, I twist some threads of this book together to invite you to practice disabling and *dis*-attending, to consider anew the world's disclosures and their dispersal in your everyday experiences. Remember, how and whether the sensory input that we process in any given moment materializes disability are shaped by the diffractions among disabled and dominant *dis*-attentions circulating around us as well as our own practices of *dis*-attending. Disability's emergence is likewise shaped by our attention to constructions and experiences of race, gender, queerness, and socioeconomic status; it is shaped by the cultural behaviors and practices embedded in the environments we navigate; it is shaped by our own histories and by how others around us collectively attend; and it is shaped by particular times and places and by particular configurations and material arrangements. The stories we tell are active participants in how disability comes to presence and how we come to perceive disability. These perceptions are themselves shaped by how stories come to us as well as their materiality.

I will share two stories below—one taken from an interview with a disabled faculty member and another published in an academic essay. As you read, consider how they have come to you and maybe how they came to be included in this epilogue. Notice what signs of disability I and their tellers include and what their tellers, or I, might be eliding or *dis*-attending. You, my readers, will perceive different details in these scenes than I do. What are they?

"I'm Getting Old"

This story comes as Nicola, a white contingent faculty member with a chronic illness, describes various masking strategies she uses to ensure that her disability is not recognized by her students or colleagues. She tells this story during a spoken interview with a research interviewer who openly identifies as disabled.[1] Nicola explains to the interviewer that one way she masks her disability is to use her material environment. For instance, she makes sure that she is always close to a desk or a wall while teaching so that if she experiences weakness in her legs, she can casually lean against them to support herself. She also adopts particular behaviors to distract attention from manifestations of her disability. For instance, when she loses her grip and whatever she is holding slips from her hands (e.g., a piece of chalk), she will just wave it off as if she cannot be bothered. As she shared these examples, she included a detailed account of how she—on the first day of class—prepares her students to notice various signs of disability:[2]

> So (0.7), at the beginning of the semester, uh ((*smiles*)) (1.3), I usually just tell them, you know listen (0.5), I'm getting old, and they <u>love</u> that because they always think I (mean) you know I look young, I'm young and I look even younger than I am, so listen guys, listen, I'm getting old (1.0), so, I need you to bear with me cause it's gonna take me a few weeks to learn your names, but ((*adjusts glasses*)) (1.0), I want you to know that, this is <u>not</u> because I don't care about you, I <u>very much</u> want to learn your names (1.0), it's just that, you know, you start getting old ((*chuckles*)).[3]

In this story, there is no immediately obvious, yellow diamond-shaped sign loudly announcing "Disabled Person in Area," but Nicola does make some incongruous juxtapositions. One such juxtaposition comes as she tells her students, "I'm getting old," a line she repeats three times in the quotation above. She directly connects "I'm getting old" with telling her students that it will take her time to learn their names. She goes on to stress to her students that "this is <u>not</u> because I don't care about you, I <u>very much</u> want to learn your names (1.0) it's just that, you know, you start getting old ((*chuckles*))." When Nicola confesses that she won't learn her students' names quickly, she cues in to information that she assumes her students are likely to perceive or learn from her as the term proceeds, and she works to deflect a potential interpretation they might make—that her not knowing their names is a sign of disinterest or lack of care.

A second juxtaposition emerges in the discrepancy between Nicola's physical appearance and her claims about aging. In an aside to the interviewer, Nicola explains that her students "<u>love</u> that because they always think I (mean) you know I look young, I'm young and I look even younger than I am." So another sign of disability here is that gap, that space between "I'm getting old" and Nicola's youthful appearance. For many this incongruity may be resolved as being a joke and is likely why her students "love that": it taps into humor as a way of getting the class to go along with the fact that their teacher is not going to know their names right away. Recall here Friedman's work showing that inconsistent or ambiguous information tends to get filtered out of active perception rather than being resolved or incorporated into a new understanding. For many perceivers, it is easier to ignore these contradictions and go along with Nicola's cheerful assertion of aging and age-related decline than to materialize disability.

It is important to note how differently Nicola talks about these signs of disability with the interviewer than with her students. As Nicola narrates her chronic illness during her interview, she uses her stories to contextualize accounts of what happens in her classroom. For instance, she narrates for the interviewer the nature and disabling effects of her chronic illness (e.g., "I have, my short term memory is, is, quite poor"; "I have a very big lesion, in my frontal lobe"), and she attaches value and meaning to her disability and how it matters to her self-presentation in the classroom, explaining that not being able to learn her students' names quickly "kind of upsets me (0.8), because (1.0), I (0.5), take, I've always taken pride in the fact that I, care about my students, like it's something that's, in my statement of teaching philosophy, is that, one of the things that I do, is that I make an effort to, connect with my students (0.5), and (0.5), help them understand, that I truly care about them, that I'm really committed to their success and this is part, of my pedagogy is that I connect with my students as human, beings."[4] In her storying, Nicola uses these strategies to cue her listeners—the disabled researcher participating in the interview scene as well as me writing this epilogue and you reading it—to notice the signs of disability in her story and to *dis*-attend to them by moving them into active awareness rather than letting them be backgrounded or elided by other frames.

"I Need an Accessible Classroom"

Let me turn now to a second example, this one composed for publication in an academic essay collection. In "Risking Experience: Disability, Precarity, and Disclosure," Kate Kaul, a middle-aged, white contingent faculty member, relates an exchange with a university administrator as she requests a room change due to an inaccessible classroom. The administrator insists on a disclosure from someone in the class before being willing to schedule an accessible classroom. Kaul finally gives in:

"Ok," I say. "I need an accessible classroom. I need it for me. I need it because I have a disability that makes it hard for me to go up and down stairs. And I need to be able to reach the AV equipment." That may have seemed irrelevant but in another new disability studies course that year, for another new department, I had been surprised to find the AV console was welded to the wall, halfway up a flight of steep concrete steps. It hadn't occurred to me that I couldn't operate an AV console positioned at shoulder height, with my feet on different steps, until I gave it a try.

There's another pause. I'm confused; I thought I had given the administrator what she needed. But she tells me, "I'm going to need a thing."

"A thing?"

"A . . . thing."

"What kind of thing?"

"A letter from a doctor?"

An image flashes through my mind of the kind of letter my family doctor—a good sport in so many ways—might write that would set out the reasons why the disability studies course in the summer session of a mostly-newly built university should be held in a room the students and the instructor can be expected to get into. It's long and angry and it looks a bit like a paper I once wrote. I put it down for now.

"I can get one," I concede. "But I also have this thing." I hoist my foot up on to the arm of the chair I've been standing next to, peel up the leg of my—cropped—trousers (it is, after all, the summer term), and point out the plastic brace. I can't believe she hasn't seen it before. She sees it now.

"Oh, of course," she says. "If they ask . . ."

"I'll get the thing," I finish.

But they don't.

At home, my girlfriend laughs: "Good thing you wore your splints today!"[5]

Kaul's story highlights the absurdity around what is readily recognized as disability and the dominant *dis*-attentions that lead the administrator to filter out her splint until called to notice it in the context of a disability accommodation request. Kaul's analysis calls out some of the dominant *dis*-attentions circulating in this scene: that disability is visible; that even "invisible disability" can be legibly disclosed and made perceptible; and "that an unfortunate individual (because those AFOs are very uncomfortable, especially the right one) brings disability to a classroom that was fine until she turned up."[6] Yet, at the same time, Kaul argues, "showing someone a brace, an AFO, is not really disclosing, is it? In some ways, it's misdirection." Drawing on Tanya Titchkosky in *The Question of Access*, Kaul notes that an accessible classroom "is not just a space. It is a matter of timing, of priority (and hierarchy), of communication, of legibility, recognition, imagination. . . . In an accessible room, by which I mean, one where I can use all of the things that I need in order to teach, I may not have to disclose my disability to my students."[7]

Kaul's desire for an environment that does not compel disclosure is an important one. Classroom disclosures occur amidst academic hierarchies that almost always give first consideration to tenured faculty in terms of course assignments, schedules, and classrooms and least consideration to those contingent faculty most likely to be experiencing disability and academic precarity. Too, such disclosures are often compelled within bureaucratic negotiations infused with asymmetries of power and control that mandate how and when disability—or any claims to identity or experience for that matter—must be made legible.

In *Counterstory*, Aja Martinez relates an episode involving a human resources clerk and a form that she needed to fill out before starting a new faculty position. Preparing to go in and fill out the form, Martinez writes, "Returning to the emphasis on the concept of being *human*, in this body that is societally raced, gendered, and aged, among other things, and when thinking about access for this body in university spaces with buildings that, for all intents and purposes, look like Hogwarts, I believed—and my use of the past tense here is intentional—I believed that on the days I want to be treated like the PhD and professor that I am, I needed to 'dress the part.'"[8]

So the next day, she puts on professional attire, drives an hour to her campus to complete this form, and is relieved when she arrives and overhears another person, a white man, apparently there for the same reason she is. However, when she gets to the desk, instead of a smooth interaction, the HR employee questions Martinez skeptically: "Are you employed here?" When Martinez finally asks, "Do I need to produce my school ID?" the administrator gives Martinez a dismissive hand gesture and indicates she should fill out the form in a nearby waiting area. When Martinez returns with the completed form, the administrator questions her again: "Is this *your* school ID number?" This bureaucratic skepticism when juxtaposed with Kaul's pointing out her splints highlights the complex intersections of embodied legibility that shape how disability is disclosed and made available for perception.

Making Bodies Available for Perception

The two stories shared above and the various forms of textual mobility that have enabled them to arrive here, in front of you right now, highlight several tensions and juxtapositions around disability's materialization in everyday textual encounters. For instance, both Nicola's and Kaul's accounts demonstrate the impact that contingent employment in academia can have on embodied perception and perceptibility. They each highlight risks associated with making one's body available for others to fully perceive. The degree to which Nicola can highlight to the interviewer how she works to ensure that others will filter out signs pointing to disability is shaped by the material conditions and environment of the interview. Both Kaul and Nicola highlight different intersections of embodied privilege, particularly when juxtaposed against other accounts, such as Martinez's, that ask questions about who can assume and in what contexts that others will take their disclosures seriously as raced, gendered, and classed disorientations intra-act. These accounts also emphasize the changing dynamics of access, moving at different times, speeds, places, spaces, environments, and intra-actions.

They also consider questions about how stories come to move and take shape within particular contexts. Nicola's accounts, like Tonia's in chapter 3, were recorded as part of a research interview. In the course of listening to and engaging these accounts, I have decontextualized these stories from their original emergence and recontextualized them here in this book. Kaul's and Martinez's accounts first emerged in texts written for publication and are being recirculated within this book. Each of the texts' original material forms mattered for how they came to existence and how they came to me. Their emergence in this book is shaped by this text's material forms as well as my own authorial body and the intra-actions that have led me to compose in this place, at this time. Your engagement with these accounts and how they matter to your own practices of *dis*-attention and disabling is the culmination of a life lived to this point and the possibilities that open up (and close off) through this engagement. What I have shared here are not the only—or even necessarily the most important—disorientations for continuing to meander among and engage with signs of disability, and one of my hopes for this book is for it to motivate (or unmotivate) other intra-acting possibilities.

Some Disabling Prompts

- What are the signs of disability that you notice in the stories that come to you? In the stories that you tell?
- What forms of dominant and disabled *dis*-attentions enable and/or elide the materialization of disability? How do they intra-act with one another, creating different diffraction patterns?
- How does the world's materiality disclose to you? What are these disclosures and what can you learn from them?
- Where and how do you make efforts to participate in processes of disabling? Where and how do you notice disabling around you? Where and how do disabled *dis*-attentions intra-act?[9]
- Where and how do dominant and disabled *dis*-attentions, disclosures, and practices of disabling circulate, get amplified, gain resonance, and participate in the ongoing dynamics of intra-action?

I hope that you will take these questions and help us all learn new practices of attention that center disability's intra-acting emergence and open up possibilities for radical inclusion and entanglement among disabled *dis*-attentions.

ACKNOWLEDGMENTS

Many readers spent time with parts of the manuscript over the years I was writing it, and they have all helped shape the words on this page, although any faults are my own.

I am grateful to audiences who engaged with versions of this project through classroom visits, colloquia, brown-bag lunches, and public lectures over the course of my working on this book. Engaged and interactive listeners at Appalachian State University, Columbia University, Eastern Michigan University, Georgetown University, Kansas State University, Michigan State University, Montclair State University, the National Center for Institutional Diversity at the University of Michigan, New Mexico State University, Northern State University, Washington State University, Wayne State University, the University of Arizona, the University of California–Berkeley, the University of California–Santa Cruz, the University of Illinois–Urbana-Champaign, the University of Maryland, the University of Michigan UMinDS program, the University of Nebraska-Lincoln, the University of Notre Dame, the University of Toledo, the University of Washington–Seattle, the University of Wisconsin–Madison, and the University of Wisconsin–Milwaukee were valuable interlocutors as the project germinated.

Thanks to all the readers who read and gave feedback on various parts of the manuscript: Allyson Day, Rebecca Dingo, Jessica Edwards, John Ernest, Asia Friedman, Anne Gere, Naomi Greyser, Kate Kaul, Caitlin Larracey, Travis Chi Wing Lau, Maren Linett, Kathleen Lyons, Elisabeth Miller, Peter Mortensen, Clare Mullaney, Therí Alyce Pickens, Jessica Restaino, Stephanie Rosen, Rebecca Sanchez, Mary Schleppegrell, Jamie Sutherland, Meg Sweeney, Sara Webb-Sunderhaus, Remi Yergeau, and Sean Zdenek. Especial thanks to the manuscript readers who visited Delaware and interacted with an early draft of the book as part of a manuscript review sponsored by my department: Jay Dolmage, Michael Hames-García, Jai Virdi, and Julian Yates. Asia Friedman generously read a complete draft of the book and helped me think more critically about perception. My BIMR writing group, Bethany Davila, Katie Gindlesparger, Amy Reed, and Shannon Walters, have looked at more versions of some of the chapters than I can count and been an enduring source of encouragement while I was writing, and Katie read the entire book cover to cover as I prepared the manuscript for submission.

Two anonymous reviewers for New York University Press, and a third reviewer from the University of Michigan Press, provided essential critical perspective and commentary on the book. Ellen Samuels's never-failing enthusiasm for the project from its early stages was a big factor in influencing me to work with New York University Press because of the way she understood the project and the questions I wanted to pursue in it. I am grateful to series editors Michael Bérubé, Robert McRuer, and Ellen Samuels as well as New York University Press editor-in-chief Eric Zinner for believing in the work. Thanks to Furqan Sayeed and Jonathan Greenberg for helping clarify many aspects of the publication process, and to Jay Dolmage for his support in making arguments for simultaneous print and OA publication.

Every single person who has taken or shared photographs of signs with me has informed my thinking on this project. Thanks to Tara Wood and Aimi Hamraie for allowing me to use some of their images in this book or in work that led to this book, and to Peter Mortensen, who generously prowled the UIUC campus for additional photographs and did some digging into campus signage. Thanks to Kristin Lindgren and Kaitlyn Delaney, whose images of yellow diamond-shaped signs appear in chapter 2. Many, many other people have also shared images, stopped their cars in weird places, or gone out of their way to take photographs, and every single one of these contributions has helped me better understand the genre of yellow diamond-shaped signs.

I am fortunate to have been able to write with Lauren Rosenberg while working on this book. My thinking on *dis*-attention was sharpened through work we did together in writing "Entanglements of Literacy Studies and Disability Studies," *College English* 83, no. 4 (2021): 261–88, which received the 2021 Richard Ohmann Outstanding Article in *College English* Award from the National Council of Teachers of English.

Margaret Price collaborated with me to interview disabled faculty, and I am grateful for all that I learned about accessible interviewing in that process, as well as for the ways her work is transforming higher education. Janel Atlas, Carolyne King, and Megan O'Donnell produced rough transcripts for each interview involving aural data as well as collaborated in transcript theorizing and experimentation. Andrew Ferris formatted the book's citations and bibliography when I submitted the full manuscript, and John Clements provided final proofreading, citation checking, and copyediting.

This project could not have been completed without support for the research and writing provided by an American Association of University Women Postdoctoral Fellowship, the Conference on College Composition and Communication Research Initiative, the National Center for Institutional Diversity at the University of Michigan, the University of Delaware College of Arts and Sciences, the University of Delaware General University Research Grant program, the University of Delaware President's Diversity Initiative, the University of Delaware Interdisciplinary Humanities Research Center, the University of Delaware Disability Support Services Office, and the University of Delaware Center for the Study of Diversity.

In acknowledging the various forms of financial and material support I received in writing this book, I want to particularly recognize the opportunity afforded by a 2019–20 scholar-in-residence position with the National Center for Institutional Diversity, during which I was able to complete a great deal of generative thinking and work on this book. Tabbye Chavous, Ching-Yune Sylvester, Marie Ting, and Dana Brown all provided essential support for infrastructures for faculty writing and community building. I am grateful to Urmitapa Dutta and W. Carson Byrd for being scholars-in-residence with me, and to the University of Michigan Departments of Psychology (especially Jacqueline Mattis) and English (especially David Porter and Remi Yergeau) for sponsoring my time in Michigan. Without the generosity of a bedroom in Remi Yergeau's house and its proximity to a twenty-four-hour doughnut shop for only the cost of splitting the utilities and groceries, I could not have afforded to accept this fellowship—an underrecognized aspect of the privilege and the costs involved in being able to write and think for a year with institutional sponsorship.

Just as NCID offered a wonderful space to germinate thinking and writing, so too did UD's Center for the Study of Diversity create space, connection, and opportunities for intellectual connection that helped sustain this project over the years I spent in Delaware. James M. Jones and Rosalie Rolón-Dow, along with other CSD faculty, were early sponsors of this work, along with Maggie Andersen, former vice provost for faculty affairs and diversity at Delaware.

I owe a huge debt to UD's amazing Interlibrary Loan staff, led by the intrepid Megan Gaffney, whose efforts were especially vital when the COVID-19 pandemic closed down access to facilities and ILL staff members helped maintain access to innumerable resources.

Many colleagues at the University of Delaware offered various forms of camaraderie and support that provided the fertile ground necessary for germinating long-term thinking and projects: Steve Amendum, Maggie Andersen, Robin Andreasen, Deb Bieler, Nicolette Bragg, Pascha Bueno-Hansen, Pam Cook, Celeste Doaks, Heather Doty, Mary Bowden, Jessica Edwards, Laura Eisenman, John Ernest, Dawn Fallik, Peter Feng, Asia Friedman, Gabrielle Foreman, Megan Gaffney, Colette Gaiter, Jennifer Gallo-Fox, Meg Grotti, Laura Helton, Carol Henderson, Theresa Hessey, Elizabeth Higginbotham, Lindsay Hoffman, Melissa Ianetta, James M. Jones, Jessica Jones, Megan Killian, Jenny Lambe, Ed Larkin, Ikram Masmoudi, Claire McCabe, Jennifer McConnell, Meg McGuire, Devon Miller-Duggan, Shailen Mishra, Kristen Poole, Andy Ross, Jennifer Saylor, Tim Spaulding, Ben Stanley, Dana Veron, Sarah Wasserman, George Watson, David Wilson, Miranda Wilson, Regina Wright, Julian Yates, and Sean Zdenek. Underneath all of these collaborations and connections was a foundation provided by Kaylee Olney and Ann Marie Green, who smoothed many aspects of faculty life and made the department a wonderful place to work for thirteen years.

Many of my brand-new University of Washington colleagues have welcomed me into the department and provided generous community as I completed the final stages of the book: Anis Bawarshi, Carolyn Busch, Eva Cherniavsky, Stephanie Clare, Rush Daniel, Annee Fisher, Amanda Friz, Juan Guerra, Jacob Huebsch, Habiba Ibrahim, Douglas Ishii (through Facebook no less!), Michelle Liu, Colette Moore, Suhanthie Motha, Candice Rai, Cristina Sánchez-Martín, Neil Simpkins, Holly Shelton, Sumyat Thu, Karla Tofte, Josie Walwema, and Joanne Woiak.

Thanks to my fellow deaf academics who have engaged draft paragraphs and shared insight across different deaf experiences, participated in problem-solving and masterminding activities, supported me and others when we needed to vent frustration or get perspective, and cheered achievements big and small. Huge thanks to Nomy Bitman, Teresa Blankmeyer Burke, Jill Bradbury, Brenda Brueggemann, Janine Butler, Linda Campbell, Ana Caicedo, Mel Chua, Michele Cooke, Alina Engelman, Margaret Fink, Michele Friedner, Kristen Johnson, Sara Halpern, Kristen Harmon, Dahlys Hoot, Krista Kennedy, Christopher Krentz, Maren Linett, Alex Lu, Jennifer Nelson, Alison O'Daniel, Holly Pearson, Rebecca Sanchez, Alma Schrage, Carrie Solomon, Tonya Stremlau, Jessi Ulmer, Jai Virdi, Christian Vogler, KT Wagner, Mel Whalen, Thomas Wright, and Manako Yabe for all the ways they have contributed to this community over the years.

My fellow Badasses in Mid Rank have provided necessary encouragement and cheer at many points over the course of writing, and especial thanks to the colleagues who have shared space with me at various write-on-sites, physical and virtual, over the last decade. Write-on-sites remain one of my very favorite writing accountability strategies: writing in the company of others never fails to give me a sense of calm and a commitment to showing up and doing the work on a daily basis. In particular a Virtual Write-on-Site, first nudged in the early months of the COVID-19 pandemic by Ikram Masmoudi and currently maintained by Jenn Fishman, kept me together and showing up day after day even in the early, terrifyingly uncertain days of the pandemic, and they made writing in the morning in my bathrobe with fresh coffee feel like curling up with a warm blanket.

Like write-on-sites, writing retreats have come to be an essential part of my writing process, especially for working through some of the big, complicated ideas in this project. Every person I have shared writing retreat space with is somewhere in this book: I can remember where I was when particular parts took shape and who I was sharing space with during those moments. Eternal gratitude and love to Jacquie and Nadine Mattis, who have created a magical space at Easton's Nook in Newark, New Jersey, for supporting writers and writing, sustaining body and spirit and creating space for the writing to flow, and to Michelle Boyd at Inkwell Academic Writing Retreats, who first cued me on to Easton's Nook and whose subsequent messaging and newsletters have helped me understand what writing retreats might look like or be.

Nadia Brown, Joan Furey, Jen Gallo-Fox, and Mark Robinson were essential to so, so, so many stages of this project, from the early days of gathering research and figuring out what this book was even going to be about to the long, hard slog of being in the middle of a really big project, when I often felt unsure the project would even come to completion. Regular late-night pandemic conversations with Jenn Fishman and Lauren Rosenberg kept us all laughing when we really needed some levity in our lives. Shelaswau Crier, Naomi Levy, and Kirsten Rodine-Hardy offered early writing-buddy accountability support, and this book would have been much harder to write without the weekly masterminding and (almost-)annual writing retreat spaces I have been able to share with Sheri Breen, Estela Ene and Sarah Rivett.

As I hope is evident in the pages of this book, the DS-RhetComp colleagues who first invited me into disability studies, and the many people who have sustained this community over the years, are one of the biggest reasons I am here today. Too, the broader disability studies community outside of writing studies catalyzed my efforts to build a perceptual apparatus attuned to disability and has helped me learn to shift and grow in needed (and sometimes painful) ways. They have participated in many conference encounters, coffee chats, social media exchanges, emails, mentoring outreach, and much more, and every time I tried to create even a partial list, my fears of who I might forget stopped me from trying to make a full accounting—if you have interacted with me in any of these spaces, please know that you are part of this book.

Finally, biggest everything to the people who have made it possible for me to write, thrive, and love: my parents, Holly and Dick Kerschbaum, my in-laws, Debra and Whitney Sutherland, and my family, Jamie, Rosemary, and Rhys.

An earlier version of part of chapter 2 appeared in "Signs of Disability, Disclosing," *enculturation* 30 (2019), http://enculturation.net/.

APPENDIX

Disabled Faculty Study Materials

RECRUITMENT EMAIL
Subject: Interview Study: Faculty Members
with Disabilities in Higher Education
From: Kerschbaum, Stephanie L <kersch@udel.edu>

Date: Wed 5/15/2013 1:00 PM

To: DEAFACADEMICS LISTSERV
(cross-posted to DS-HUM, SDS, Disabled
Academics, Deaf Academics, and
DS-RhetComp)

Dear Colleagues,
We are conducting a study to understand faculty members' experiences
with disability disclosure in higher education settings. This study is
IRB-approved, with the University of Delaware serving as the IRB of
record.

As part of this study, we will interview faculty members at a variety
of higher education institutions, in different disciplines and areas of
study, and from all ranks and types of faculty employment, and we are
recruiting interested participants who would be willing to be interviewed about their experiences negotiating disability in academe. The
remainder of this letter provides a brief overview of what we might
ask of you should you be interested in participating, and gives you an
avenue for contacting us to ask further questions.

The first stage involves completing a brief questionnaire asking for demographic and biographical information in order to help us determine

our interview pool ([survey link]). We will use this information to help us achieve diversity sampling and thus include a broad range of experiences, positions, and intersectional attributes in our study.

We estimate that this survey, administered via Survey Monkey, will take less than five minutes to complete. Your responses will not be anonymous, but all information from this survey will be kept confidential and only available via password-protected Survey Monkey account to the two researchers conducting this study—Stephanie Kerschbaum and Margaret Price. Results of this survey will be used for sampling purposes only; they will not be analyzed as part of the interview data. We will destroy survey responses when sampling for the interview study is complete.

The second stage of our project, should you be selected as part of our sample, will involve an interview in which we will ask you about your experiences negotiating disability in academe. In keeping with our aim of conducting "accessible interviews," interviews will be conducted in participants' and researchers' preferred modalities, ranging from in-person to Skype to internet-messaging to asynchronous email exchanges. One of the questions on our introductory survey will ask you to identify your preferred means of participating in an interview.

If you have any questions, please contact us using the information below. If you have questions related to the IRB process, please contact the University of Delaware Institutional Review Board at [phone number] or via email at [email address].

Warmly,

Stephanie Kerschbaum, [email address and phone number] (text only)

Margaret Price, [email address and phone number] (voice or text)

Stephanie L. Kerschbaum, Ph.D.

Assistant Professor, Department of English

Faculty Scholar, Center for the Study of Diversity

University of Delaware

[mailing address]

[faculty web site]

[link to Disability Disclosure in/and Higher Education Conference web site]

RECRUITMENT SURVEY

We are asking you to complete this brief demographic survey to help us select interview participants for a research study focused on disability disclosure by faculty members. This project is IRB-approved, with the University of Delaware serving as IRB of record.

This information is for study participant selection only and will not be analyzed or reported in any way. Responses will be destroyed after interview participants have been selected.

1. Please tell us your name, academic position, department or program, and the primary institution you work at.
2. Do you work full-time or part-time? If "other," please describe.
3. What is your teaching, research and service load? Describe in a way that makes sense to you (hours per week, percentages of job description, or other).
4. Institution type (Please choose based on your primary place of employment)
   - Comprehensive/Regional Institution
   - Liberal Arts College
   - Research University
   - Community College
   - Other (please specify)
5. What is the nature of your disability? Feel free to explain this however you prefer.
6. What is your gender and/or sex? Please add any explanation or qualification needed. More than one choice can be selected.
   - Female
   - Male
   - Genderqueer
   - Transgender
   - Other
7. What is your age?
   - 20 or younger
   - 21–30
   - 31–40
   - 41–50

- 51–60
- 61–70
- 71–80
- 81–90
- 91+

8. What is your racial and/or ethnic identification? Please add any explanation or qualification needed. More than one choice can be selected.
   - Black/African-American
   - Latino/a
   - American Indian
   - Asian-American
   - International (non-US citizenship)
   - White
   - Other

9. What would be your preferred modality(ies) for an interview? Select as many as you would like.
   - In-person (Researchers will travel to you, or we will meet in a mutually convenient place, such as an academic conference or other venue.)
   - Telephone
   - Skype
   - E-mail
   - Internet-messaging (e.g., AIM or G-chat)

10. What is the best way for us to contact you? If you indicate a phone number, please mention whether you prefer text messaging or voice as well as the best times to contact you, including your time zone.

INTERVIEW PROTOCOL

Each semistructured interview involved four central questions aimed at extracting narratives about interviewees' experiences with disability and faculty life.

1) What is your name, title, and primary place of work?
2) Have you ever discussed your disability at work? If yes, tell me about a time when you've done that. Invite details and context.

If no, ask why not; tell me about situations where you have avoided addressing or raising your disability at work.

3) Tell me about the environment you work in (e.g., office space, daily routines, schedules, expectations, locations, materials and technologies used)

4) What specific accommodations do you have in place?

5) Are there accommodations you wish you could have, but don't?

NOTES

INTRODUCTION

1 Barad, *Meeting the Universe Halfway*, 185.

2 See Kerschbaum, "On Rhetorical Agency and Disclosing Disability in Academic Writing."

3 For more on some of my job market experiences, see Brueggemann and Kerschbaum, "Disability"; Dolmage and Kerschbaum, "Wanted."

4 Here is an example, this one created for the 2014 National Women's Studies Association Conference:

> Dear _____,
>
> I write to introduce myself to those of you who don't know me, to smile and wave at those who do know me, as well as to express my plans to attend your NWSA panel, "TITLE" (I hope I've found everyone's correct email addresses; if I've gotten any email addresses wrong, please do forward to the correct ones—I'm relying on google searches and university directories, which are not always up to date, to get this information :-))
>
> I'm excited to learn a lot during your panel. As I know some of you already know, I am deaf, and will have interpreters with me at the conference. Because it is very hard for interpreters to keep up with rapidly-delivered conference presentations using often-unfamiliar academic vocabulary, it is important to me to be able to read along with a hard copy of any scripted remarks you plan to read or share. This is particularly important for this particular conference because only two interpreters have been contracted for the duration of my time at the conference, and thus, I want to save their primary interpreting energy for unscripted moments at the conference (e.g., session Q&As, ad-libbing or off-script moments during talks).
>
> As you've likely noticed, the NWSA has urged presenters to bring additional copies of their papers as an accessibility move (LINK to NWSA website): "Speakers are asked to bring five copies of their papers, even in draft form, for the use of members who wish to follow the written text. Speakers who use handouts should prepare some copies in a large-print format (Sans-serif font, 16-point type size). Speakers should indicate whether they want their papers and handouts returned."
>
> At least one person in your audience (me!) will need this accommodation, and the interpreters will need a copy as well so that they can follow

along and help me keep up with where the presentation is, and so that they know when they may need to interpret a digression or something that is ad-libbed during the presentation.

There are a couple of ways that this has worked for me in the past:

—sometimes people want to email me the paper ahead of time (and I can print my own copy to bring for myself and the interpreters). There may still be other people in the audience who would benefit from reading the paper, however.

—usually, people print additional copies before leaving for the conference, while acknowledging that revisions may happen during the plane flight or just before the presentation. In the past, I have had people verbally acknowledge that they are skipping parts of their script (e.g., "I'm going to move now to the top of page 5, if you're following along on my script"). It is no big deal at all for the script to have slight differences from the presented paper.

—sometimes people are able to print additional copies of their talk at the conference itself by using the hotel business center or at a nearby Kinko's or copy center.

If you want your paper returned, that is no problem and usually people write that on the first page of their script, something along the lines of "Script made available for accessibility purposes only, please return at end of presentation."

Again, I'm looking forward to the conference and excited to see/meet you.

Warmly,

Stephanie Kerschbaum

5 These experiences directly led to and shaped my thinking around "multimodal inhospitality," a concept I developed in "Multimodality in Motion." Yergeau et al., "Multimodality in Motion."

6 Blankmeyer Burke, "Choosing Accommodations." For more on the complexities of academic interpreting, see also ASL Core, "Home: ASLCORE"; Blankmeyer Burke and Nicodemus, "Coming out of the Hard of Hearing Closet"; and Hauser, Finch, and Hauser, eds., *Deaf Professionals and Designated Interpreters.*

7 See Hubrig and Osorio, eds., "Enacting a Culture of Access in Our Conference Spaces."

8 Kerschbaum, *Toward a New Rhetoric of Difference,* chapter 2.

9 According to H-Dirksen Bauman, "As soon as the orthographic proclamation of 'big D' Deaf was made, Deaf Studies scholars had to describe what made someone Deaf as opposed to deaf," and no one has yet resolved it. First suggested by James Woodward in a 1972 course he was teaching, it has been taken up in largely reductive ways that often suggest there is a clear distinction between the terms. That it has remained problematic to pin down and define has perhaps contributed to its continued disproportionate influence. As Rebecca Sanchez (personal

communication) pointed out, "Part of what rankles about d/D is it not only pro-
duces a false binary, but that it centers a certain kind of understanding about what
identity is (stable, fixed, internal to the individual) that seems to totally miss the
relational/orientational stuff that (to me anyway) is so vital to understanding what
deafness is/how it means." While Michele Friedner has usefully complicated some
of the tensions in d/Deaf through Foucault's conceptions of biopower and subject
formation as she notes that claiming and negotiating between these identifications
and communities can involve both acts of oppression and acts of resistance, it
still seems to require too much containment and explanation to be fully useful.
In this, I am particularly entranced with Brenda Jo Brueggemann's critique of it
in theorizing "betweenity." Brueggemann notes the frequency with which copy
editors and others in mainstream spaces—largely hearing audiences—keep asking for this refrain, this explanation, a definition that we can easily and readily
point to. But, she says, "What if we stop footnoting and explaining and educating
them—meaning largely hearing people—again and again and again? For almost
thirty years now, we've learned to chant, from almost rote memorization, when
we explain the 'difference' between little d and big D deafness. But they never
seem to hear a word about any of this, and so we go on footnoting and explaining
and educating about the distinctions between 'Deaf' and 'deaf.'" Brueggemann's
observation that hearing people never seem to hear this distinction or understand it points to ways that this discourse has solidified, rather than remaining
malleable and interesting. The result is a situation in which many participants in a
Deaf Academics Facebook group that I am part of express complex relationships
to naming themselves as deaf or associating with a broader community of deaf
people. Such a conversation can only happen among recognition of the complexity of negotiations around deafness, and it is my hope for this book—and the
framework of signs of disability—to open up new possibilities for understanding
deafness as a capacious onto-epistemological category that resonates with more
people. Bauman, "Introduction," 9; Friedner, "Biopower, Biosociality, and Community Formation"; Brueggemann, *Deaf Subjects*, 14–15.
10 Samuels, *Fantasies of Identification.*
11 See also Lindquist, *A Place to Stand.*
12 See Kerschbaum and Price, "Centering Disability in Qualitative Interviewing,"
102–3, for more on this interviewing situation.
13 Fink, "Disabling Research Methods"; Garrison, "Theorizing Lip Reading as Interface Design."
14 Hamraie and Fritsch, "Crip Technoscience Manifesto."
15 Lukin, "Science Fiction, Affect, and Crip Self-Invention."
16 Ferguson, *The Reorder of Things.*
17 Minich, "Enabling Whom?"
18 Siebers, "Returning the Social to the Social Model."
19 Kerschbaum, *Toward a New Rhetoric of Difference*, 67.
20 Kimmerer, *Braiding Sweetgrass*, 40–41.

21 Kimmerer, *Braiding Sweetgrass*, 46.

22 Barad, *Meeting the Universe Halfway*, 33.

23 Barad, *Meeting the Universe Halfway*, 151.

24 Barad, *Meeting the Universe Halfway*, 67.

25 Barad, *Meeting the Universe Halfway*, 207.

26 Barad, *Meeting the Universe Halfway*, 133.

27 Barad, *Meeting the Universe Halfway*, 207.

28 Cedillo, "What Does It Mean to Move?"; Hsu, "Reflection as Relationality"; King, Gubele, and Anderson, *Survivance, Sovereignty, and Story*; Martinez, *Counterstory*; McKittrick, *Dear Science and Other Stories*; Malea Powell, "Rhetorics of Survivance: How American Indians Use Writing." *College Composition and Communication* 53, no. 3 (2002): 396–434; Powell, "Listening to Ghosts"; Powell et al., "Our Story Begins Here"; Riley-Mukavetz, "Developing a Relational Scholarly Practice"; Titchkosky, *The Question of Access*; Villanueva, *Bootstraps*; Villanueva, "Memoria Is a Friend of Ours"; Yergeau, *Authoring Autism*.

29 Shomura, "Exploring the Promise of New Materialisms."

30 Barad, *Meeting the Universe Halfway*, 149.

31 Barad, *Meeting the Universe Halfway*, 149.

32 "ASL Sign for DISABILITY," Sign Language ASL Dictionary, accessed January 25, 2021, https://www.handspeak.com/; "Elective Disability," ALSCORE, Rochester Institute of Technology, accessed January 25, 2021, https://aslcore.org/.

33 "ASL Sign for DEAF," Sign Language ASL Dictionary, accessed January 25, 2021, https://www.handspeak.com/.

34 "ASL Sign for BLIND," Sign Language ASL Dictionary, accessed January 25, 2021, https://www.handspeak.com/.

35 "ASL Sign for WHEELCHAIR," Sign Language ASL Dictionary, accessed January 25, 2021, https://www.handspeak.com/.

36 The term "bodymind" has been developed by Margaret Price as a feminist materialist disability concept. As she explains, "Because mental and physical processes not only affect each other but also give rise to each other—that is, because they tend to act as one, even though they are conventionally understood as two—it makes more sense to refer to them together, in a single term" (269). Price, "The Bodymind Problem and the Possibilities of Pain." See also Schalk's *Bodyminds Reimagined*.

37 Price, "The Bodymind Problem and the Possibilities of Pain."

38 Yergeau, *Authoring Autism*, 193. On betweenity, see Brueggemann, *Deaf Subjects*.

39 Clare, *Brilliant Imperfection*; Kafer, *Feminist, Queer, Crip*; Kim, *Curative Violence*; Jaipreet Virdi, *Hearing Happiness*.

40 Pickens, *New Body Politics*, chapter 1.

41 Sanchez, *Deafening Modernism*, 151.

42 See e.g., Bamberg, "Positioning between Structure and Performance"; Georgakopoulou, *Small Stories, Interaction, and Identities*; Labov and Waletzky, "Narrative Analysis"; Ochs and Capps, *Living Narrative*; Wortham, *Narratives in Action*.

43 Vidali, "Disabling Writing Program Administration"; Yergeau, "Disable All the Things."
44 Kerschbaum, "On Rhetorical Agency and Disclosing Disability in Academic Writing."
45 Kerschbaum, "Anecdotal Relations."

CHAPTER 1. *DIS*-ATTENDING

1 "Americans with Disabilities Act (ADA)," University of Michigan, accessed January 24, 2021, https://lsa.umich.edu. Another account of negotiating the accommodation process at U-M was shared by Remi Yergeau:

> Upon arriving on campus as a new assistant professor, I begin searching for information on how to request disability accommodations. To my surprise, there is nothing that I can find about this online. The campus disability services office only serves students. The hospital's autism center only serves individuals under the age of twenty-five. The university HR website might as well be the seventh circle of hell. Photos of shiny happy presumably able people holding hands in a cubicle. Who smiles in an HR cubicle? Are they holding hands because they need a love contract? Whither disability policy? Disabled faculty and staff seem not to exist.
>
> In desperate need of disability support, I make several inquiries. I ask my new colleagues about who the disability services contact is for faculty, and one colleague tells me there's no such thing. I am eventually routed to the mother of a friend who used to TA at my university fifteen years ago, who then routes me to an administrative assistant, who then routes me to a singular name at HR: The university's ADA coordinator, whose office is located on another campus in a lonely administrative building near the football stadium. I take two city buses to get there. The ADA coordinator is lovely, kind, welcoming. She asks what I need. I describe the accommodations I received at my previous institution and she stops me. "I don't grant requests," she explains. "I mediate disputes over requests." I need to contact my chair and/or direct supervisors, she tells me. I need to request accommodations from the body that, in part, determines whether or not I receive tenure.

Yergeau, "Creating a Culture of Access in Writing Program Administration," 160–61.

2 See Blankmeyer Burke, "Choosing Accommodations"; Blankmeyer Burke and Nicodemus, "Coming out of the Hard of Hearing Closet."

3 See, for instance, Brown and Leigh, eds., *Ableism in Academia*; Kerschbaum, Eisenman, and Jones, eds., *Negotiating Disability*; Price, "Time Harms"; Price et al., "Disclosure of Mental Disability by College and University Faculty"; Vance, ed., *Disabled Faculty and Staff in a Disabling Society*.

4 Dolmage, *Academic Ableism*.

5 Bell, "Introducing White Disability Studies."

6 See, for instance, work by Nirmala Erevelles, especially her book *Disability and Difference in Global Contexts*, as well as the transformative work done under the

umbrella of DisCrit, a subfield of educational research that links disability studies and critical race theory. Connor, Ferri, and Annama, eds., *DisCrit*; Erevelles, *Disability and Difference in Global Contexts*.

7 Schalk and Kim, "Integrating Race, Transforming Feminist Disability Studies."

8 Ahmed, *Queer Phenomenology*.

9 *Oxford English Dictionary*, s.v. "dis-, prefix," accessed January 22, 2020, https://www.oed.com/.

10 Virdi, "Materializing User Identities through Disability Technologies."

11 Williamson, *Accessible America*.

12 See Sanchez, "'Human Bodies Are Words'"; Friedner and Helmreich, "Sound Studies Meets Deaf Studies"; Garrison, "Theorizing Lip Reading and Interface Design"; Fink, "Disabling Research Methods."

13 E.g., Hammer, *Blindness through the Looking Glass*; Ceraso, "Sound Never Tasted So Good"; Ceraso, *Sounding Composition*; Bivens, "Rhetorical Ventriloquism, Earwitnessing, and Soundscapes in a Neonatal Intensive Care Unit (NICU)"; and Campt, *Listening to Images*.

14 Manning et al., "Affective Attunement in an Age of Catastrophe."

15 Siebers, *Disability Theory*. See also Canguilhem, *The Normal and the Pathological*; Dolmage, *Disability Rhetoric*; and Davis, *Enforcing Normalcy*.

16 Puar, *The Right to Maim*.

17 Chen, *Animacies*.

18 Bérubé, *The Secret Life of Stories*; Linett, *Bodies of Modernism*; Rodas, *Autistic Disturbances*; and Sanchez, *Deafening Modernism*.

19 This was one of the ways my experience at Michigan was dramatically different from my encounters on many other campuses, where the question of cost is often a primary barrier to access provision (see Hubrig and Osorio). But cost was still a central factor animating the interactions I had, given that NCID's budget, as a small center on campus, did not have the flexibility to simply take on the full cost of my accommodation needs. Scott Lissner and many others have long advocated for centralized models for funding disability accommodation so that this important institutional need is not disproportionately borne by specific individuals or entities but is shared across the campus. It was this decentralized model that required me, supported by NCID, to work to get other units to participate in—at least by paying for—accommodations at their events. Hubrig and Osorio, eds., "Enacting a Culture of Access in Our Conference Spaces."

20 This resource continues to be circulated across U-M's campus, and as of Spring 2021 was linked on several websites and in active use even though I had completed my scholar-in-residence in Spring 2020. This point underscores the lack of centralized attention to access knowledge, which is effectively being crowdsourced at Michigan by units and individuals who add pieces of information and resources here and there.

21 I have heard story after story of deaf undergraduates arguing and fighting to get the colleges and universities they attended to build effective accommodation

structures that enabled their access to learning environments. I took my interpreting access at Ohio State for granted, but the ease with which I was able to get it has been far from the norm for many deaf college students.

22 Schnitzer and Dede, *Diversity Includes Disability*.

23 Hamraie, *Building Access*. I discuss access knowledge in more detail in chapter 3.

24 Konrad, "Access Fatigue." The concept of microaggressions, a term that has now moved into common parlance, was first coined by Chester Pierce in 1970 and further developed in the mid-2000s by psychologist Derald Wing Sue and colleagues in talking about everyday experiences with race. Numerous scholars and writers have recognized the utility of this term in relation to other marginalized experiences, but it remains important to center the concept's racialized origins as well as to understand the interrelationships among different forms of microaggressions, including those that may seem to be disability focused but also often have racist, misogynist, and sexist resonances. Sue et al., "Racial Microaggressions in Everyday Life."

25 Barad, *Meeting the Universe Halfway*, 33.

26 Pickens, *Black Madness*, 17.

27 Pickens, *Black Madness*, 27.

28 Pickens, *Black Madness*, 29.

29 Barad, *Meeting the Universe Halfway*, 261.

30 Barad, *Meeting the Universe Halfway*, 261.

31 Barad, *Meeting the Universe Halfway*, 67.

32 Pickens, *Black Madness*, 72–73.

33 Barad, *Meeting the Universe Halfway*, 106–15. See also discussion of this concept in Mitchell, Antebi, and Snyder's introduction to *The Matter of Disability* using the example of a blind person and a white cane: the person can focus on the cane, assessing its weight and properties, or the person can use the cane to perceive their environment, but they cannot simultaneously zero in on the cane's properties *and* use it to measure (determine properties) of their surroundings. "Introduction," in *The Matter of Disability*.

34 Pickens, *Black Madness*, 73.

35 Barad, *Meeting the Universe Halfway*, 208.

36 Barad, *Meeting the Universe Halfway*, 247.

37 Barad, *Meeting the Universe Halfway*, 242.

38 Pickens, *Black Madness*, 9.

39 Hames-García, *Identity Complex*.

40 Valentine, *Imagining Transgender*, 100, emphasis in original.

41 Brune and Wilson, eds., *Disability and Passing*; Hobbs, *A Chosen Exile*; Godfrey and Young, eds., *Neo-Passing*; Kennedy, "'I Forgot I'm Deaf!'"; Samuels, "Passing, Coming Out, and Other Magical Acts"; Siebers, *Disability Theory*; Sánchez and Schlossberg, eds., *Passing*; Wald, *Crossing the Line*.

42 Siebers, *Disability Theory*.

43 Yoshino, *Covering*.

44 Samuels, "My Body, My Closet."

45 Snorton, *Black on Both Sides*, 84.

46 Snorton, *Black on Both Sides*, 14.

47 Lee and Ahtone, "Land-Grab Universities."

48 Dolmage, *Academic Ableism*, 45 (italics added).

49 Ahmed, *Queer Phenomenology*, 133.

50 Dolmage, *Academic Ableism*, 70.

51 I include image descriptions of each photograph for accessibility purposes, but also because these descriptions serve an analytic function within the chapter. Throughout, I follow guidelines for image descriptions offered by accessibility resources such as WebAIM and AbilityNet. This means I focus on "describ[ing] the information, not the picture" (Rule 2, "Five Golden Rules"). In this way, the descriptions are not intended to serve as a "neutral" recounting of what is in the image (indeed, neutrality in image descriptions is impossible, as what we notice, and consequently describe, is always influenced by what we are poised to notice). Grantham, "The Five Golden Rules of alt-text"; WebAIM: Web Accessibility in Mind, accessed January 29, 2020, https://webaim.org/.

52 This icon signifies differently depending on its context: when appearing in isolation it may be read as ungendered but when appearing alongside a female-presenting one, as male. This mutability of gender as well as the implications of extending what is a "male" icon to represent all-gender is important, especially in the context of the ISA's ungenderedness.

53 Stephanie Rosen, accessibility strategist and librarian for disability studies at the U-M libraries, made this comment on an earlier version of this chapter:

> You might also be interested to know, and not surprised to learn, that [creating and maintaining signage] is also somewhat decentralized at U-M. For example at the Library we actually have staff focused on the design of interior spaces and wayfinding, and we did some focus groups a while back with folks who use gender-neutral and/or accessible bathrooms (because in our spaces those are often the same, single-stall bathrooms) in order to redesign our signage and language, help people find their way to the bathrooms they need, and also to re-educate staff so everyone knows where they are. We then added some signage, supplemental to the required signage, to help with wayfinding to bathrooms that people need. But this only affects our main library buildings, not much relative to the whole campus, and [is] not the same as other buildings nearby.

54 Brekhus, *Culture and Cognition*.

55 Zerubavel, *Taken for Granted*, 22.

56 Friedman, *Blind to Sameness*, 33.

57 Friedman, *Blind to Sameness*, 86.

58 Friedman, *Blind to Sameness*, 86.

59 See, e.g., Banaji and Greenwald, *Blindspot*, xi.

60 Friedman, "Cultural Blind Spots and Blind Fields."

61 See, e.g., Adams, *Sideshow U.S.A.*; Garland-Thomson, *Staring*; Bogdan, with Elks and Knoll, *Picturing Disability*; Dolmage, "Framing Disability, Developing Race."

62 Vidali, "Seeing What We Know."

63 Friedman, "Cultural Blind Spots and Blind Fields," 13.

64 Brian Massumi's notion of differential attunement especially highlights the way that people experience environments, ecologies, and interactions in highly differentiated ways that are consequential for subsequent materializations and interactions. Manning et al., "Affective Attunement."

65 Ceraso, *Sounding Composition*; see also Katz, "Is There a Right Way to Be Deaf?"; Kennedy, "'I Forgot I'm Deaf!'"; and Virdi, *Hearing Happiness*, as recent examples of deaf people writing about cyborg/relations to deafness/hearing aids.

66 See Kennedy, "'I Forgot I'm Deaf!'"

67 Recall my frequent experience of being introduced with various disability and deaf euphemisms. These terms suggest to me a reluctance to say "deaf" or a fear of causing offense. And indeed, it is true that for some deaf people, deafness is dis-associated with disability. For them, deafness should not materialize disability, but rather, a cultural identity (see, e.g., Baynton; Bauman and Murray). So, the hearing aids simultaneously materialize disability—they provide me a shortcut to disclosure, as when I can just gesture toward my hearing aids while asking someone to repeat something or make sure they are looking at me. They also provide sensory input that others may perceive and/or attend as they interact with me. But whether they function as signs of disability, whether disability materializes, is a matter of carefully attending to intra-actions, perceptual apparatuses, and emergent phenomena that consequently influence subsequent intra-actions, apparatuses, and phenomena in a continual process. Baynton, *Forbidden Signs*; Bauman and Murray, eds., "Deaf Gain: An Introduction," in *Deaf Gain*.

68 Zdenek, *Reading Sounds*.

69 See Downey, *Closed Captioning*, 231–33.

70 Vanessa is my oldest friend. We met when I was in second grade and she was in third, and even though I moved to another town a year later, we have kept in touch our whole lives and still talk regularly. She is not deaf, but her dad was knowledgeable about electronics and willing to figure out how to hook up our caption decoder box. Before we started actually moving the decoder box back and forth, we rented lots of foreign films with English-language subtitles, something that continues to make us laugh every time we remember some of the films we watched. These were real, material consequences that were shaped by myriad factors that materialized some possibilities at some moments and not others. And they have persisted today, in showing me at a very early age that it was possible for hearing people—Vanessa and her network of friends, who became my friends as well through my time spent staying over at her house—to care deeply about whether or not one deaf person in their midst could watch TV with them. As I have thought about and tried to write this book, I have returned often to that

friendship and how important it has been in anchoring my own emerging and developing sense of self even as an adult, thirty-five years later.

71 See Zdenek, *Reading Sounds*; Reeb, "[This Closed Captioning Is Brought to You by Compulsive Heterosexuality/Able-Bodiedness]."

72 Cooper, *The Animal Who Writes*, see chapter 5.

73 In the work I do with faculty mentoring, I often talk with people experiencing moments of transition—moving from one institution to another or one career stage to another or navigating new professional challenges, including many embodied and health-related changes. Being continually confronted with the new and different requires differently active perceptual processes at work, and those processes happen in different ways over time as people build greater familiarity (although not always comfort) with their everyday environment.

74 Friedman, "Cultural Blind Spots and Blind Fields," 6.

75 Friedman, "Cultural Blind Spots and Blind Fields," 7.

76 I develop this more fully in Kerschbaum, "Exploring Discomfort Using Markers of Difference."

77 Zerubavel, *Hidden in Plain Sight*.

78 Friedman, "Cultural Blind Spots and Blind Fields," 8.

79 Friedman, "Cultural Blind Spots and Blind Fields," 13.

CHAPTER 2. DISCLOSING

1 Hekman, *The Material of Knowledge*, 92.

2 Price, "Un/Shared Space."

3 Titchkosky, *The Question of Access*.

4 Siebers, *Disability Theory*, 51.

5 Vidali, "The Biggest Little Ways toward Access."

6 See Dolmage, *Academic Ableism*, chapter 1, on the steep steps metaphor for academia.

7 See Dolmage, *Academic Ableism*, chapter 2, on the retrofit.

8 See Savitz, *Wheelchair Champions*.

9 "Illini Adapted Athletics Introduction," University of Illinois at Urbana-Champaign, accessed January 14, 2021, https://www.disability.illinois.edu/.

10 Guffey, *Designing Disability*.

11 Ben-Moshe and Powell, "Sign of Our Times?"

12 Hendren, "An Icon Is a Verb."

13 Fritsch, "The Neoliberal Circulation of Affects."

14 Titchkosky, *The Question of Access*.

15 Kafer, *Feminist, Queer, Crip*; Clare, *Brilliant Imperfection*; Al Zidjaly, *Disability, Discourse and Technology*.

16 The Accessible Icon Project, accessed January 14, 2021, http://accessibleicon.org/.

17 Kerschbaum, "Disabled Faculty and Linguistic Agency."

18 See Morrison, "(Un)Reasonable, (Un)Necessary, and (In)Appropriate," for a similar critique of institutional accommodation processes designed or presented

as singular moments of disclosure that subsequently resolve the question of disabled-or-not.

19 I first forward this framework in Kerschbaum, "On Rhetorical Agency and Disclosing Disability in Academic Writing."

20 Sanchez, "Doing Disability with Others."

21 Stremlau, "Deaf Pedestrians."

22 Dougher, "How Not to Be a Dick to a Deaf Person."

23 Sanchez, "Doing Disability with Others," 218.

24 Siebers explains complex embodiment as "the reciprocal transformation between the body and its environment—a reciprocity that provides for change in each term within an otherwise constant equation, the content of which is embodied and thus known in and as the body." Through complex embodiment, disabled bodyminds have immense value because it is through their experiences that they build new knowledge. Rosemarie Garland-Thomson's notion of "misfitting" likewise suggests that it is experiences of having one's body and mind "misfit" with an environment that produce knowledge as identity and subjectivity materialize through "perpetual, complex encounters between embodied variation and environments." Siebers, "Returning the Social to the Social Model," 39–48; Garland-Thomson, "Misfits."

25 Hekman, *Material of Knowledge*, 91.

26 Hekman, *Material of Knowledge*, 91.

27 Samuels, *Fantasies of Identification*.

28 Sanchez, "Doing Disability with Others," 214.

29 Sanchez, "Doing Disability with Others," 213.

30 Sanchez, "Doing Disability with Others," 213–14.

31 After publishing an early version of this chapter as Kerschbaum, "Signs of Disability, Disclosing," I received the following note from a reader:

> Our Massachusetts family sign language program instructor emphasized that we "must" get these signs as she was hit by a car when she was young. I did not think twice and we diligently made the request to the town. It was not until the signs went up, the sole signs that said Deaf Child Area, that I felt like there were arrows and flashing lights surrounding our house; calling us out as the house of the Deaf child . . . a Deaf child lives here . . . hey world, take note! And I hated the Hollywood aspect of it. So I asked the town to add the Drive Slowly signs, giving explanation for WHY the deaf child signs were there in the first place. We did not want to be spectacles. We only wanted drivers to slow down and pay attention.

32 Friedman, *Blind to Sameness*, 26.

33 Hamraie and Fritsch, "Crip Technoscience Manifesto," 2.

34 See, e.g., Abdelhadi, "Addressing the Criminalization of Disability from a Disability Justice Perspective"; Elman, "Policing at the Synapse"; Moore et al., "Accountable Reporting on Disability, Race, and Police Violence"; Sanchez, "Linguistic Othering"; Vest, "What Doesn't Kill You."

35 Titchkosky, *The Question of Access*, 73–75.

36 Friedman, "Cultural Blind Spots and Blind Fields," 8.

37 I am estimating its disappearance as happening sometime during 2016. However, much as with its appearance, I don't know when it disappeared nor when it formally stopped being part of my immediate perceptual terrain.

38 Relatedly, I have a few examples of signs that are not yellow, such as a white rectangular sign with red lettering that says, "Caution Disabled Pedestrians in Area," photographed in Newark, Delaware.

39 Some require certification of disability; others simply ask a set of questions about desired sign placement. Some indicate an age cap, and most stipulate that if the person for whom the sign is being placed moves away, residents should request that the sign be taken down. Some offer some guidelines for when a sign would be considered. Language for the signs varies from community to community as well, reflecting the variety in the signs that I have collected.

40 Some additional discussion may be important on this point, simply because of the sheer number of times this question has come up as I have presented and shared this work in different contexts. Perhaps the most common questions I get are, "Tell me more about how these signs even get placed in this environment? How did that sign get there? Who was responsible?" The truth is that I do not have access to the interactions that lead these signs to be placed in communities, although I have engaged with some of the texts that support the signs' emergence: news articles, blog posts, online forms for requesting a sign's placement. And yet, even though I *am* intensely interested in social interaction, which has been the focus of a great deal of my earlier work, this project does not rely on recordings of everyday interactions involving disclosure (for complex methodological reasons, some of which are detailed in this book's introduction). My focus on storying, then, means that I am less concerned with how a sign got there and more concerned with what sense people make—through narrative—of a sign that is in place.

41 Kuusisto, "Intersection," 80–82.

42 Dunn, *The Social Psychology of Disability*.

43 One example of this sort of expecting—and which turns up the volume on *dis*-attentions whereby disability is unexpected and thus rarely accounted for within behavioral patterns—involves people who begin interacting with me without realizing that I am deaf. A not-uncommon response is for people to get angry or perceptibly annoyed in these encounters, perhaps because I am not responding to them or perhaps because they think I am ignoring them. This is a significant source of what several opinion pieces and blogs have called "ableist anxiety" or "deaf anxiety" in my own life. Anticipating such tensions involves considerations of how, in what ways, and with what behaviors disability becomes apparent. See, e.g., Khalifa, "Deaf Anxiety."

44 Doubek, "Oklahoma City Police Fatally Shoot Deaf Man Despite Yells of 'He Can't Hear'"; Sanchez, "Linguistic Othering."

45 See also work being done by Black activists as well as racially minoritized, queer, and disabled activists in protesting and resisting police brutality and incarceration practices that are exceptionally harmful toward disabled people, and particularly Black disabled people. Ben-Moshe, Chapman, and Carey, *Disability Incarcerated*; Harriet Tubman Collective, "Disability Solidarity"; Lewis, "Stolen Bodies, Criminalized Minds, and Diagnosed Dissent."

46 Emil B. Towner acknowledges the difference in experience between navigating warning signs in a familiar environment versus experiencing signs in an unfamiliar environment (e.g., a vacation locale). Research on perception, routine, ritual, and cognitive processing has shown that as people build familiarity in their environment and in their daily practices, they attend less carefully to individual steps and moments along the way. The same goes for warning signs: perhaps when the signs are new, they are carefully attended. After a period of time, they become part of the background and are not actively perceived and attended to. Towner, "Danger in Public Spaces."

47 WisDOT Research & Library Unit, "Effectiveness of 'Children at Play' Warning Signs."

48 E.g., Brownlee, "City Reverses Stance on 'Deaf Child' Signage."

49 I have examples of each of these signs.

50 For instance, many "Keep Kids Alive, Drive 25" signs are white rectangles with black and red text and images, rather than yellow diamond-shaped caution signs.

51 Chen, *Animacies*, 24.

52 Chen, *Animacies*, 23–34.

53 Chen, *Animacies*, 55.

54 Chen, *Animacies*, 95.

55 Garland-Thomson, *Extraordinary Bodies*.

56 Chen, *Animacies*, 40.

57 Taylor, *Beasts of Burden*, 52.

58 The persistence of rhetorics that dehumanize autism are powerfully documented in Yergeau, *Authoring Autism*.

59 This is perhaps partly an artifact of the fact that during most of the writing of this book and collecting of signs, I lived in Newark, a small suburban town in Delaware, but there are also differences in how signage is placed and how people move in more densely populated urban locations that do not as readily support such signs' emplacement.

60 Taylor, *Beasts of Burden*, 59.

61 Taylor, *Beasts of Burden*, 52–53.

62 Hekman, *The Material of Knowledge*, 92.

63 Kim, "Unbecoming Human."

64 Mills, "Materializing Race," 34.

65 Johnson and McRuer, "Cripistemologies."

66 Bauman and Murray, eds., *Deaf Gain*. However, I should note that while they praise the collection, Yergeau has critiqued a troubling undercurrent of neoliberal

valuation of human difference within its chapters. Yergeau, *Authoring Autism*, 180–81.

67 Siebers, "Returning the Social to the Social Model," 42.

68 See Pickens, *Black Madness*, for a useful overview; see also Johnson, *Too Late to Die Young*.

69 Chen, *Animacies*; McKittrick, "Yours in the Intellectual Struggle"; Mitchell and Snyder, "Posthumanist T4 Memory"; Pickens, *Black Madness*; Taylor, *Beasts of Burden*; in disability rhetoric the question of speech has been a particularly fraught tension—see Bascom, ed., *Loud Hands*; Brueggemann, *Lend Me Your Ear*; Dolmage, *Disability Rhetoric*; Yergeau, *Authoring Autism*.

70 Sins Invalid, *Skin, Tooth, and Bone*.

71 Wong, ed., *Disability Visibility*; Wong, Disability Visibility Project.

72 Piepzna-Samarasinha, *Care Work*.

73 Lewis, "Stolen Bodies"; Talila T.L. Lewis, in community with Disabled Black and other negatively racialized people, especially Dustin Gibson, "January 2021 Working Definition of Ableism."

74 Ahmed, *Queer Phenomenology*, 137.

75 Barad, *Meeting the Universe Halfway*, 149.

76 Kim, "Unbecoming Human," 315.

77 Barad, *Meeting the Universe Halfway*, 185.

78 See, e.g., Chen, *Animacies*; Glick, *Infrahumanisms*.

79 Barad, *Meeting the Universe Halfway*, 377.

80 Cooper, *The Animal Who Writes*, 143.

81 Barad, *Meeting the Universe Halfway*, 396.

82 I have written about such solidifying in discussing Ann Jurecic's attention to autism as well as the deployment of disability in rhetoric and composition theorizing. Kerschbaum, *Toward a New Rhetoric of Difference*, chapter 2; Kerschbaum, "Anecdotal Relations."

CHAPTER 3. DISABLING

1 Vidali, "Disabling Writing Program Administration"; Yergeau "Creating a Culture of Access in Writing Program Administration"; Brueggemann, "An Enabling Pedagogy," 795.

2 Vidali, "Disabling Writing Program Administration," 33.

3 Minich, "Enabling Whom?"

4 Minich, "Enabling Whom?"

5 Gumbs writes,

> The survival of Black feminist intellectuals, which happens within or without the academy, is our intentional living with the memory of May Ayim's suicide after being in a mental institution; our living with the knowledge that as Audre Lorde's archival papers prove, she was denied medical leave, had to turn down prestigious fellowships (including the senior fellowship at Cornell) that required residency in places too cold for her to live during her fight

against cancer. The English Department at Hunter, which recently honored Lorde with a conference 20 years after her death, rejected her proposals at the end of her life to teach on a limited residency basis that would allow her to teach poetry intensive classes for students during warm weather in New York and to live in warmer climates during the winter based on her health needs.

Gumbs, "The Shape of My Impact."

6 Kim, "Toward a Crip-of-Color Critique."

7 Kim, "Unbecoming Human."

8 To give one example: at one academic conference, I worked to get a copy of a written script for the evening's big keynote lecture after being told the organizers could not afford to provide interpreting. I paid to print the talk at my hotel, took a shuttle to the conference location, and got settled in my seat just in time for the auditorium to plunge into darkness with only a spotlight on the presenter. I could not see the paper in front of me, much less read the script.

9 When I first arrived at Delaware I was stunned by the difference in approach taken by the interpreting agencies that the university regularly contracted with, and the approach taken by the interpreting agency I worked with in my first job at Texas A&M University. When I began at TAMU, the owner of the interpreting agency the university contracted with took me out to lunch and asked a series of questions about me, my access needs, my signing skills and preferences, and more. With this information, she worked to identify interpreters who would be a good fit for me, and she regularly and proactively communicated about various compromises and questions that came up in her efforts. This exceptionally positive experience thus set me up to be unpleasantly surprised by what felt like an approach at Delaware that was more focused on putting any warm body, regardless of fit or qualifications, into interpreting situations that for me, were high stakes professionally. Having an unqualified interpreter in my classroom, for instance, or during meetings that included my department chair, made me seem incompetent given that no one else in the room could assess what the interpreter was doing much less recognize that they were not effectively interpreting. This situation was the outcome of a complex set of local and state factors, including laws and regulations around sign language interpreting in Delaware, Pennsylvania, and Maryland; UD's geographic location in a small town that also featured the Delaware School for the Deaf; and imbalances in interpreter supply and demand, and it took years to build a local pool of high-quality interpreters who were skilled at the particular kind of academic transliteration I needed, as well as a relatively smooth process for making accommodation requests and securing interpreters for them.

10 See chapter 1, end note 6.

11 Hamraie, *Building Access*, 5.

12 Piepzna-Samarasinha, "How Disabled Mutual Aid Is Different Than Abled Mutual Aid."

13 Hamraie, *Building Access*, 115.

14 Blankmeyer Burke, "Teresa Blankmeyer Burke."

15 Krista Kennedy has written about the shifts emerging in her behavior and orientations to the world through changes in interactions with other deaf people as well as with experimenting with how often and long she wore her hearing aids. See Kennedy, "'I Forgot I'm Deaf!'"; Kennedy, "Being Seen Deaf."

16 Piepzna-Samarasinha, *Care Work*, 33.

17 Wong, Disability Visibility Project.

18 Each of the interviews conducted for this study happened at a specific moment in time, through specific material configurations, and involved different environmental surrounds. In turn, all of the interviewees shared stories that were relevant and momentous at the specific time interviews were conducted. In writing about these accounts, then, I follow Joshua Kupetz's example in adopting a convention from literary studies of orienting to each of these narratives, and the interview moment, in the present tense despite the fact that years have passed between the interviews and the writing of this book, and none of the participants are in the same situation(s) they described in their interviews. Kupetz, "Disability Ecology and the Rematerialization of Literary Disability Studies."

19 Tonia interview, September 11, 2015, segment 7. At this point let me make some notes on transcription and quoting from interviews. Each interview was divided into segments according to topic shifts. I gave each segment a title that referenced its central concept or theme. Within each segment, interview data was further subdivided into narrative episodes. Tonia's interview, for instance, was ninety-one minutes long and divided into forty-three segments. Segments ranged widely in length and number of narrative episodes. Lines in transcripts were broken when speakers took a breath or paused for less than half a second. Numbers in parentheses reflect pauses longer than half a second. Colons indicate when a sound was elongated, with more colons indicating a longer sound. Underlines indicate words that are spoken at a louder volume than surrounding speech, while degree signs indicate words spoken more softly than surrounding speech. Brackets indicate simultaneous speech, and equals signs indicate latched speech, such that there is no pause between the latched utterances. A word or question mark in parentheses indicates uncertain transcription. Paralinguistic and nonlinguistic cues are italicized and placed inside double parentheses. These transcript conventions are developed from Jeffersonian style, with the difference that I do not include auditory elements that I cannot perceive even with my hearing aid amplification, such as changes in pitch or intonation. The conventions for transcription used here are very much a product of me as a researcher and what I am poised to attend to in collaboration with research assistants who produced the first transcripts. Working from the first pass at transcription, I fine-tuned and added necessary detail through careful listening and relistening.

When quoting from transcripts within the text, I make the following modifications: line breaks are indicated with commas, and I do not include interviewer interjections and backchannel utterances in quotations unless they figure directly into the analysis. In a similar vein, I also delete brackets indicating overlapping speech as well as equals signs indicating latched speech unless I am attending to the inter-actional dynamics of the utterance in the analysis. Sacks, Schegloff, and Jefferson, "A Simplest Systematics for the Organization of Turn-Taking for Conversation."

20 Barad, *Meeting the Universe Halfway*, 185.

21 I have written about this at the end of chapter 3 of *Toward a New Rhetoric of Difference*, as well as in "Exploring Discomfort Using Markers of Difference."

22 See appendix for recruitment email, demographic survey, and semistructured interview protocol.

23 While there is not space in this chapter to fully explore differences across interview modalities, it is nevertheless the case that the interview space was—in every case—meaningful for the narratives that emerged during interviews. The two interviews that I conducted using instant messaging made this particularly apparent to me. In one, the time it took to conduct our conversation over instant message led us to divide the interview into two two-hour-long sessions held months apart, and our second session ended up focusing on how questions asked during the first led the interviewee to move forward with a formal accommodation request. A second example involved my realization that the pace of my typing and my learned practice of backchannel cueing that I had developed over years of regularly using IM to chat with friends and colleagues (e.g., typing "nodding" to indicate when I was physically nodding) seemed to distract the interviewee, leading me to practice waiting, rather than proactively forwarding information about what I was doing in the IM space.

24 Price, *Mad at School*, 204–11. See also Price, "Disability Studies Methodology."

25 For more detailed discussion of this study's approach to accessible interviewing, see Kerschbaum and Price, "Centering Disability in Qualitative Interviewing," as well as Price and Kerschbaum, "Stories of Methodology." A similar ethic shaped Chapple, Bridwell, and Gray's approach to interviewing in "Exploring Intersectional Identity in Black Deaf Women."

26 Barton, "Further Contributions from the Ethical Turn in Composition/Rhetoric," 599.

27 See Friedman, *Blind to Sameness*; Zerubavel, *Taken for Granted*.

28 See Baker-Bell, "For Loretta"; Benjamin, Donovan, and Moody, "Sacrifices, Sister-hood, and Success in the Ivory Tower"; Gumbs, "The Shape of My Impact"; Nam, "Making Visible the Dead Bodies in the Room."

29 Disabled faculty who had experienced significant transitions were particularly poised to highlight how signs of disability signified in different ways and de-scribed different factors that influenced their experiences of disability in different situations. These transitions included—but were not limited to—changing institutions, earning or being denied promotion and/or tenure, experiencing traumatic or stressful events, teaching new or different classes, undergoing new research projects (especially those that involved moving into disability-related topics), experiencing changes in their disability status or experience (such as the

emergence of new symptoms, health improvement, deteriorating health/abilities, gaining or losing allies or support systems), undergoing often protracted struggles for access and accommodation in different professional spheres, and experiencing new or different accommodations. As I wrote this chapter, examples from across the interview data readily and routinely emerged as relevant for showcasing additional disclosures enacted by signs of disability as well as disability's emergence as a phenomenon. However, moving across interview examples required a more distanced analytic stance than the one I am most interested in developing here.

30 Some caveats are important to mention here. My encounters with Tonia encompassed her responses to the recruitment survey, several email exchanges, and a phone interview lasting just over ninety minutes. It was important to me as a researcher that I respect participants' time and boundaries around research involvement, so I adhered carefully to participants' expressed desires regarding interview follow-ups and continued interaction. This means that while there are numerous details that I wish I had followed up on in the interview or that I could do continued member-checking on as I wrote, Tonia's wishes mean that my analysis and discussion here is limited to what she shared in this interview and this interview's unfolding at a specific moment in time as part of a particular material configuration. It further means that I choose to err on the side of caution in revealing potentially identifying details, and I work to not assume knowledge beyond what Tonia communicated in our research exchanges.

31 Tonia interview, segment 7.

32 Tonia interview, segment 5.

33 Bailey, *Misogynoir Transformed*, 1. See also Bailey and Trudy, "On Misogynoir."

34 Bailey, *Misogynoir Transformed*, 12.

35 Wortham, *Narratives in Action*, 19.

36 Tonia interview, segment 7, lines 22–25.

37 Tonia interview, segment 7, lines 38–39.

38 Tonia interview, segment 7, lines 42–49.

39 Tonia interview, segment 7, lines 56–57.

40 Tonia interview, segment 8.

41 Alcoff, *Visible Identities*, 188.

42 Alcoff, *Visible Identities*, 188.

43 Ahmed, *Queer Phenomenology*, 131.

44 Kahneman, *Thinking, Fast and Slow*.

45 Mills, "Materializing Race," 36.

46 Bailey and Mobley, "Work in the Intersections," 29.

47 Bailey, "Misogynoir in Medical Media"; Bailey, *Misogynoir Transformed*; Bailey and Trudy, "On Misogynoir."

48 Bailey, "Misogynoir in Medical Media," 2.

49 Hitt, *Rhetorics of Overcoming*, 18–19. See also Linton, *Claiming Disability*.

50 Tanya Titchkosky talks about "taking a leave" as a primary response to disability in *Question of Access*.

51 See Konrad, "Reimagining Work"; Konrad, "Access Fatigue."

52 Tonia interview, segment 8.

53 Tonia interview, segment 15. For more on the ADA see Davis, *Enabling Acts*; Goren, *Understanding the Americans with Disabilities Act.*

54 Barad, *Meeting the Universe Halfway.*

55 Zerubavel, *Taken for Granted.*

56 Schiffrin, *Discourse Markers.*

57 Schiffrin, *Discourse Markers*, 268.

58 In *Research Interviewing*, Elliot G. Mishler describes "you know" coming up as interviewees check in with interviewers to determine whether they have adequately answered the question:

> Tim Anderson (personal communication) has pointed out to me how an even more implicit response by an interviewer, namely, silence, may influence a respondent's answer. When interviewing individuals with chronic pain he asks open-ended questions about their experiences and how they cope with their problems. If he remains silent after the initial response, neither explicitly acknowledging or commenting on the answer nor proceeding immediately to a next question, respondents tend to hesitate, show signs of searching for something else to say, and usually continue with additional content. Sometimes they look for a sign that the interviewer understands or try to elicit a direct assessment with a query like, "You know?" Their "answers" are as responsive to his assessments as to the original questions. They display the respondents' effort to arrive at a shared understanding of the meaning of both questions and answers.

Mishler, *Research Interviewing*, 57.

59 Schalk and Kim, "Integrating Race, Transforming Feminist Disability Studies," 32.

60 Ahmed, *Queer Phenomenology*, 129.

61 In *Interviewing as Qualitative Research*, for instance, Irving Seidman recommends that interviewers "limit [their] own interaction," arguing that backchannel cues and evaluative comments like "right" (transcript 3.1, lines 75, 79, 120, 141, 143) and "oh jeez" (transcript 3.1, line 90), which recurred throughout Tonia's interview "run the risk of distorting how the participant responds" (90). Even as Seidman recognizes in his approach to qualitative interviewing that meaning making in interviews is "a function of the participant's interaction with the interviewer" (23), he warns against distorting the stories and data through too much interviewer interaction. Seidman, *Interviewing as Qualitative Research.*

62 See, e.g., Robillard, "Seeking Adequate Rhetorical Witnesses for Life Writing"; Wortham, "Interactional Positioning and Narrative Self-Construction."

63 Okun et al., "(Divorcing) White Supremacy Culture."

64 Margaret Price and Stephanie L. Kerschbaum, "Our Interdependent Methodology" in "Stories of Methodology."

65 Kerschbaum, in Price and Kerschbaum, "Stories of Methodology," 48–49.

66 Yergeau, "Rehabilitation ≠ what we do."

67 Konrad, "Access Fatigue."

68 See also Kerschbaum and Price, "Centering Disability"; Nusbaum and Lester, eds., *Centering Diverse Bodyminds in Critical Qualitative Inquiry*.

69 See Ahmed, *Queer Phenomenology*, especially chapter 3.

70 The cost of purchasing analytic software as well as of paying research assistants also points to my privilege as a faculty member at a public research university with access to funds to support her research. Without these funds, I could not have done this study or secured access to the materials and narratives I write about here. Deaf faculty are extremely underrepresented in public research institutions, another factor that limits the possibilities for research to be informed by and grounded in deaf onto-epistemologies. Smith and Andrews, "Deaf and Hard of Hearing Faculty in Higher Education"; Woodcock, Rohan, and Campbell, "Equitable Representation of Deaf People in Mainstream Academia."

71 I struggled with this in my first book, too, in which I had to be dragged, with extreme reluctance, to write about how my deafness shaped my approach to working with linguistic data. Kerschbaum, *Toward a New Rhetoric of Difference*, 24–25.

72 Thanks to Natasha Abner for helping me understand this point.

73 Kerschbaum, "Sign Language Transcription and Qualitative Research Methodologies."

74 Bailey, *Misogynoir*; Bailey and Trudy, "On Misogynoir."

CHAPTER 4. DISPERSING

1 Park and Bucholtz, "Public Transcripts"; Urban, "Entextualization, Replication, and Power."

2 Clare, *Exile and Pride*; Hockenberry, *Moving Violations*; Johnson, *Too Late to Die Young*; Simi Linton, *Claiming Disability*; Mairs, *Waist-High in the World*.

3 It is worth noting that such work has long been the focus of book historians, and I should acknowledge a course on Material Culture in Nineteenth Century America that I took as an undergraduate at Ohio State with Susan Williams (English) and Barbara Groseclose (History of Art), which invited precisely these kinds of questions about material objects in texts as well as texts as material objects. This course has stayed with me even as I have pursued many other paths and directions for my work.

4 Kerschbaum, "On Rhetorical Agency and Disclosing Disability in Academic Writing."

5 Friedman, *Blind to Sameness*; Zerubavel, *Taken for Granted*.

6 Titchkosky, *The Question of Access*, 50.

7 Friedman, *Blind to Sameness*, 86.

8 Schalk, *Bodyminds Reimagined*, 139.

9 Lukin, "Science Fiction, Affect, and Crip Self-Invention," 232.

10 Scholars have attended to some of these material dimensions and tensions to understand literary texts. See, for instance, Mullaney, "Dickinson, Disability, and

a Crip Editorial Practice"; Mullaney, "'Not to Discover Weakness Is the Artifice of Strength'"; Silverman, "Neurodiversity and the Revision of Book History."

11 Barad, *Meeting the Universe Halfway*, 76–77.
12 Murphy, *Sick Building Syndrome and the Problem of Uncertainty*, 1–2.
13 Canagarajah, "Weaving the Text," 17.
14 Canagarajah, "Weaving the Text," 18.
15 Vieira, "What Happens When Texts Fly," 77.
16 Flores, "Stoppage and the Racialized Rhetorics of Mobility."
17 Vieira, "What Happens When Texts Fly," 78.
18 Hints of this significance emerged through my experiences fielding questions about my deafness and its relationship to my writing. Kerschbaum, "On Rhetorical Agency and Disclosing Disability in Academic Writing."
19 Waite, *Teaching Queer*, 18.
20 Waite, *Teaching Queer*, 18.
21 Waite, *Teaching Queer*, 22.
22 The mattering of student bodies to how teachers read is reinforced in research on writing assessment that highlights how imagined and real encounters between teachers and students' bodies shape those assessments. For more on assessment and imagined bodies, see Davila, "Indexicality and 'Standard' Edited American English"; Davila, "Standard English and Colorblindness in Composition Studies"; Dryer, "At a Mirror, Darkly"; Inoue, "Racism in Writing Programs and the CWPA"; Inoue and Poe, eds., *Race and Writing Assessment*.
23 Sanchez, *Deafening Modernism*, 41–42.
24 Waite, *Teaching Queer*, 20–21.
25 Dingo, "Re-Evaluating Girls' Empowerment," 141.
26 Bell, *Walking on Fire*.
27 Dingo, "Re-Evaluating Girls' Empowerment," 143.
28 See, for instance, Hartman, "Venus in Two Acts."
29 See, for instance, Fielder and Senchyne, eds., *Against a Sharp White Background*; Samuels, *Fantasies of Identification*; and Snorton, *Black on Both Sides*.
30 Moody-Turner, "'Dear Doctor Du Bois,'" 48.
31 Elizabeth McHenry likewise considers how Black writer and activist Mary Church Terrell's archive of "failed publication" makes a case for considering the different kinds of literary access that different writers, at different times, have had or worked toward. The very fact of Terrell's unpublished writing, her extensive readership that included friends, professional acquaintances of all sorts, publishers and editors, and writing instructors, to offer only a partial list, insists that Terrell was an accomplished author despite the fact that the work that was most important to her did not reach the stage of publication. Her belief in the uses of imaginative fiction, her understanding of the workings of the publishing industry, and perhaps most impressively, her persistent critique of the "conspiracy of silence" she believed was in part to blame for her literary failure, contribute to a more nuanced understanding

of the range of literary opportunities and obstructions and the particular social and cultural situations underlying early twentieth-century African-American print culture. McHenry, "Toward a History of Access," 383–84.

32 Moody-Turner, "Dear Doctor Du Bois," 58; see also Moody-Turner, "Prospects for the Study of Anna Julia Cooper."

33 See also Brittney Cooper's theorizing from Anna Julia Cooper's work what she terms "embodied discourse," a form of "Black textual activism wherein race women assertively demand the inclusion of their bodies and, in particular, working-class bodies and Black female bodies by placing them in the texts they write and speak." Cooper, *Beyond Respectability*, 3.

34 Martinez, *Counterstory*, 20.

35 See McHenry, *Forgotten Readers*.

36 Alexander, "Materiality, Queerness, and a Theory of Desire for Writing Studies."

37 Muñoz, *Disidentifications*. For examples of work taking up Muñoz's concept of disidentification, see Egner, "'The Disability Rights Community Was Never Mine'"; Kim, "Asexuality in Disability Narratives"; Schalk, "Coming to Claim Crip."

38 Muñoz, *Disidentifications*, 93.

39 Muñoz, *Disidentifications*, 31.

40 Valentine, *Imagining Transgender*, 100, emphasis in original.

41 Cedric Burrows, in *Rhetorical Crossover*, describes material effects that occur as Black musicians move their work from predominantly Black environments into more mainstream ones.

42 Vidali, "Disabling Writing Program Administration," 37.

43 Vidali, "Disabling Writing Program Administration," 35.

44 Vidali, "Disabling Writing Program Administration," 35.

45 See Vidali, "Hysterical Again"; Vidali, "Out of Control"; and Vidali and Keedy, "Productive Chaos."

46 In an analysis of interviews with scholars about their experiences navigating academic peer review, Zachary C. Beare and Shari J. Stenberg note that in contrast to pretenure scholars, who tended to be more deferential to reviewers and editors, midcareer and senior scholars expressed less concern about negative reviewer feedback or feedback they disagreed with. Beare and Stenberg, "'Everyone Thinks It's Just Me.'"

47 Here, too, as Moody-Turner would remind us, unpublished texts and unfinished ones can also materialize disability, perhaps in their unfinishedness but also through other material dimensions.

48 Craig, "A Story-less Generation."

49 Craig, "A Story-less Generation," 17–18.

50 See Perryman-Clark and Craig, eds., *Black Perspectives in Writing Program Administration*; Craig and Perryman-Clark, "Troubling the Boundaries"; Symposium contributors Jasmine Kar Tang, Noro Andriamanalina, Sherri Craig, Collin Lamont Craig, Staci M. Perryman-Clark, Regina McManigell Grijalva, Genevieve

García de Müeller, Cedric D. Burrows, James Chase Sanchez and Tyler S. Branson, "Challenging Whiteness and/in Writing Program Administration and Writing Programs." *WPA: Writing Program Administration* 39, no. 2 (2016): 9–52; Carter-Tod and Sano-Franchini, eds., "Black Lives Matter and Anti-Racist Projects in Writing Program Administration."

51 Pickens, *Black Madness*; Bailey and Mobley, "Work in the Intersections"; Schalk and Kim, "Integrating Race, Transforming Feminist Disability Studies."

52 Kim, "Toward a Crip-of-Color Critique"; Gumbs, "The Shape of My Impact."

53 See Nishida, "Neoliberal Academia and a Critique from Disability Studies."

54 Bailey and Mobley, "Work in the Intersections," 25.

55 Bailey, "Race and Disability in the Academy."

56 Bailey and Mobley, "Work in the Intersections," 21.

57 Carmen Kynard critiques knowledge-making practices in writing studies for the way they reproduce racist logics by "not speak[ing] or writ[ing] against the ways our institutions actively reproduce inequality." Kynard, "Teaching while Black," 3.

58 Numerous signs of disability emerge across these descriptions. For instance, M. O'Brien and Cynthia Pengilly write, "We are two early-career scholar-teachers with disabling chronic health conditions: Dr. Pengilly is a cisgender Black woman who is co-director of the Online Technical Writing Program, and Dr. O'Brien is a nonbinary multiracial Tamil person who coordinates the Language and Literature Program at CWU." Carter-Tod and Sano-Franchini, eds., "Black Lives Matter and Anti-Racist Projects in Writing Program Administration."

59 Rak, *Boom!*, chapter 2.

60 Because Dewey's classification system limited topics related to Blackness to a single decimal entry, Porter intervened to reclassify many books under other categories, such as those marked for music, literature, and more. Helton explains, Dewey's 1927 index, which Porter consulted, listed these classes under "Negro": "Vocal music—Negro minstrelsy and plantation songs," "Slavery," "Education of special classes," "Negro troops in the U.S. Civil War," "the 13th and 14th Amendments," "Household personnel," "Race ethnology," "Mental characteristics as influenced by race," and "Suffrage" (*Decimal Classification and Relative Index*). For any text that did not attend to these subjects, the protocol was to place it at 325.26, a number in political science, 320, under "Colonies [and] Migration," 325, for works on "Emigrants of a special country or race," 325.2. An editorial note explained that "in United States 325.2 will relate almost wholly to specific nationalities . . . e.g., 325.26 Negro question" (*Decimal Classification and Relative Index*). Thus, nearly every object relating to African American life and history—aside from those on slavery, suffrage, minstrelsy, education, or domestic labor—landed in a section of the library reserved for works about people foreign to the nation. Helton, "On Decimals, Catalogs, and Racial Imaginaries of Reading," 101–3.

61 Helton, "On Decimals, Catalogs, and Racial Imaginaries of Reading," 101.

62 Helton, "On Decimals, Catalogs, and Racial Imaginaries of Reading," 108.

63 Helton, "On Decimals, Catalogs, and Racial Imaginaries of Reading," 112.

64 In a pair of 2015 blog posts discussing his experience figuring out how to classify transgender and disability activist Eli Clare's memoir *Exile and Pride*, Netanel Ganin found that the "options are to class it as a biography under a class of people needing 'Protection, assistance, relief'—or to place it alongside all *medical* works on the same condition," a problematic binary given the ways that medical and disability perspectives can enact disability differently. Netanel Ganin, "Disability in the Library of Congress Classification Scheme—Part 2"; see also Ganin, "Disability in the Library of Congress Classification Scheme—Part 1."

65 One example of how these logics and materials of classification matter for perceptual apparatuses—as Dorothy Porter's work emphasizes—came from Clare Mullaney, who commented on an early version of this chapter that in her archival explorations she regularly finds herself having to use pathologizing language in order to find and access disability-related materials. Such work is never neutral.

66 See, e.g., Noble, *Algorithms of Oppression*.

67 Of course, one of those challenges—which Couser acknowledges—is that those who do not recover from cancer often do not have the energy, time, and body-mind resources needed to tell those stories, often leaving it up to family members, friends, and other loved ones to fill in the gaps and tell those stories. It is in this genre that Jessica Restaino's *Surrender* fits, as Restaino accompanies a close friend, Sue Lundy Maute, through her experience with and eventual death from breast cancer. Even as it is Maute's story, shared intentionally throughout her disease and her experience of dying, it is Restaino-as-researcher-and-friend who is able to write, publish, and circulate Maute's account. Couser, *Recovering Bodies*; Restaino, *Surrender*.

68 See Rak, *Boom!*

69 Alter, "Best Sellers Sell the Best Because They're Best Sellers."

70 Allyson Day takes up this question of marketability in exploring accounts written about people's experiences with HIV+. Day notes that the stories that get most readily amplified and circulated are those that emphasize illness as an individual problem rather than as deeply intertwined with systemic, structural inequity. The result is that those who write—and publish—these accounts are rewarded not for calling out the racism, ableism, heterosexism, and sexism that shape experiences of illness but for telling accounts of individual responsibility for wellness. Day, *The Political Economy of Stigma*.

71 Here it is worth asking the question, Do we need to move disability experiences into mainstream spaces? I would argue, yes—and point to the success of *Disability Visibility* as perhaps one of the most powerful disability-centric texts published by a trade press and circulating widely among both disability communities and mainstream communities. However, it is likewise important to acknowledge the value of audiences and spaces *for* disabled people for building practices of *dis*-attention and ethical engagement that can then sustain disabled lives outside of care-based disability-centric spaces (see, e.g., Piepzna-Samarasinha, *Care Work*;

Piepzna-Samarasinha, "How Disabled Mutual Aid Is Different Than Abled Mutual Aid"). Jillian Wiese has been particularly active in critiquing the dominance of nondisabled writers writing about disability and achieving broad circulation for their work while disabled writers struggle to get recognition, reviews, and promotion for their books (see, e.g., Tullivan, "Tips for Writers by Tipsy Tullivan").

72 Crosby, *A Body, Undone*; Gay, *Hunger*; Laymon, *Heavy*; Millett-Galant, *Re-Membering*; Prahlad, *The Secret Life of a Black Aspie*; Richardson, *From PHD to PhD*; Savageau, *Out of the Crazywoods*.

73 Khakpour, *Sick*.

74 Brown, "Q&A."

75 During the writing of this chapter, a message circulated on DS-HUM (a disability-studies-in-the-humanities listserv) from someone interested in teaching Cheryl Savageau's book *Out of the Crazywoods* but concerned about its cost for students and thus asking for other suggestions. In response, another listserv poster shared a discount code that would bring the cost of the hardcover book down. Here, again, networks of information, recommendation, and resource sharing converge to make certain texts more readily available and others more difficult to procure or access. Savageau, *Out of the Crazywoods*.

76 There is an interesting tension between the mass-market accessibility of Khakpour's book and the class and economic privileges that accompany publication by a major trade publisher and that are hinted at in the stylishness of her author's photo as well as in her ability to seek treatment and relocate around the United States in doing so, making implicit claims about access to resources for maintaining her health.

77 Kleege, "Aurality," 206.

78 See Schalk and Kim, "Integrating Race, Transforming Feminist Disability Studies"; Day, *The Political Economy of Stigma*.

79 Nye, "Porochista Khakpour's *Sick*," 685.

80 Genette, *Paratexts*.

81 Schalk and Kim, "Integrating Race, Transforming Feminist Disability Studies," 38.

82 Khakpour, *Sick*.

83 In Ersula J. Ore's *Lynching*, she prefaces the book with an "Author's Note" that explains why she could not use the word "murder" to describe the state-sanctioned killings that she wrote about. Because of legal definitions of murder and the issue of publisher and authorial liability, she had to write around the word "murder"—and commit acts of linguistic violence upon herself and her readers—with her word choices. *Lynching*, xii–xvi.

84 Khakpour, *Sick*, 1.

85 Khakpour, *Sick*, 1–3.

86 Dolmage *Disability Rhetoric*, 31.

87 Dolmage, *Disability Rhetoric*, 34.

88 Khakpour, *Sick*, 1.

89 Khakpour, *Sick*, 21.

90 Thanks to Allyson Day for sharing this observation.
91 Khakpour, *Sick*, 245.
92 Clark, "Porochista Khakpour, Author of *Sick*."

EPILOGUE
1 Nicola interview, July 11, 2013. Interview conducted by Margaret Price.
2 See end note 19 attached to the first quotation from Tonia in chapter 3 for how I edited the transcripts for quoting in the manuscript.
3 Nicola interview, July 11, 2013. Interview conducted by Margaret Price.
4 Nicola interview, July 11, 2013. Interview conducted by Margaret Price.
5 Kaul, "Risking Experience."
6 Kaul, "Risking Experience," 177.
7 Kaul, "Risking Experience," 178.
8 Martinez, *Counterstory*, 106.
9 Here, I recommend Jay Dolmage's discussion (and critique) of a disability version of the Bechdel Test in *Disability Rhetoric* as well as disability activist Mia Mingus's reflections on the forces that often keep disabled people apart from each other. Dolmage, *Disability Rhetoric*, 48–49 fn 12; Mingus, "Reflections on an Opening."

BIBLIOGRAPHY

Abdelhadi, Abla. "Addressing the Criminalization of Disability from a Disability Justice Perspective: Centring the Experiences of Disabled Queer Trans Indigenous and People of Colour." *Feminist Wire*, November 21, 2013. https://thefeministwire.com/

The Accessible Icon Project, accessed January 25, 2020. http://accessibleicon.org/

Adams, Rachel. *Sideshow U.S.A.: Freaks and the American Cultural Imagination*. Chicago: University of Chicago Press, 2001.

Ahmed, Sara. *Queer Phenomenology: Orientations, Objects, Others*. Durham, NC: Duke University Press, 2006.

Al Zidjaly, Najma. *Disability, Discourse, and Technology: Agency and Inclusion in (Inter) action*. Basingstoke, Hamsphire, UK: Palgrave Macmillan, 2015.

Alcoff, Linda Martín. *Visible Identities: Race, Gender, and the Self*. New York: Oxford University Press, 2006.

Alexander, Jonathan. "Materiality, Queerness, and a Theory of Desire for Writing Studies." *College English* 83, no. 1 (2020): 7–41.

Alter, Alexandra. "Best Sellers Sell the Best Because They're Best Sellers." *New York Times*, September 19, 2020. https://www.nytimes.com/

ASL Core. "Home: ASLCORE." Rochester Institute of Technology, accessed January 24, 2020. https://aslcore.org

Bailey, Moya. "Misogynoir in Medical Media: On Caster Semenya and R. Kelly." *Catalyst: Feminism, Theory, Technoscience* 2, no. 2 (2016): 1–31.

Bailey, Moya. *Misogynoir Transformed*. New York: New York University Press, 2021.

Bailey, Moya. "Race and Disability in the Academy." *Sociological Review*, January 25, 2019. https://www.thesociologicalreview.com/

Bailey, Moya, and Izetta Autumn Mobley. "Work in the Intersections: A Black Feminist Disability Framework." *Gender and Society* 33, no. 1 (2019): 19–40.

Bailey, Moya, and Trudy. "On Misogynoir: Citation, Erasure, and Plagiarism." *Feminist Media Studies* 18, no. 4 (2018): 762–68.

Baker-Bell, April. "For Loretta: A Black Woman Literacy Scholar's Journey to Prioritizing Self-Preservation and Black Feminist–Womanist Storytelling." *Journal of Literacy Research* 49, no. 4 (2017): 526–43.

Bamberg, Michael. "Positioning between Structure and Performance." *Journal of Narrative and Life History* 7, no. 1–4 (1997): 335–42.

Banaji, Mahzarin R., and Anthony G. Greenwald. *Blindspot: Hidden Biases of Good People*. New York: Delacorte Press, 2012.

Barad, Karen. *Meeting the Universe Halfway: Quantum Physics and the Entanglement of Matter and Meaning*. Durham, NC: Duke University Press, 2007.

Barton, Ellen. "Further Contributions from the Ethical Turn in Composition/Rhetoric: Analyzing Ethics in Interaction." *College Composition and Communication* 59, no. 4 (2008): 596–632.

Bascom, Julia, ed. *Loud Hands: Autistic People, Speaking*. Washington, DC: Autistic Self-Advocacy Network, 2012.

Bauman, H-Dirksen L. "Introduction: Listening to Deaf Studies." In *Open Your Eyes: Deaf Studies Talking*, edited by H-Dirksen L. Bauman, 1–32. Minneapolis: University of Minnesota Press, 2008.

Bauman, H-Dirksen L., and Joseph J. Murray, eds. *Deaf Gain: Raising the Stakes for Human Diversity*. Minneapolis: University of Minnesota Press, 2014.

Baynton, Douglas C. *Forbidden Signs: American Culture and the Campaign against Sign Language*. Chicago: University of Chicago Press, 1996.

Beare, Zachary C., and Shari J. Stenberg, "'Everyone Thinks It's Just Me': Exploring the Emotional Dimensions of Seeking Publication." *College English* 83, no. 2 (2020): 103–26.

Bell, Beverly. *Walking on Fire: Haitian Women's Stories of Survival and Resistance*. Ithaca, NY: Cornell University Press, 2001.

Bell, Christopher M. "Introducing White Disability Studies: A Modest Proposal." In *The Disability Studies Reader*, 2nd edition, edited by Lennard J. Davis, 275–82. New York: Routledge, 2006.

Benjamin, Shanna Greene, Roxanne Donovan, and Joycelyn Moody. "Sacrifices, Sisterhood, and Success in the Ivory Tower." *CLA Journal* 60, no. 1 (2016): 84–92.

Ben-Moshe, Liat, Chris Chapman, and Alison C. Carey, eds. *Disability Incarcerated: Imprisonment and Disability in the United States and Canada*. New York: Palgrave Macmillan, 2014.

Ben-Moshe, Liat, and Justin J. W. Powell. "Sign of Our Times? Revis(it)ing the International Symbol of Access." *Disability & Sociology* 22, no. 5 (2007): 489–505.

Bérubé, Michael. *The Secret Life of Stories: From Don Quixote to Harry Potter, How Understanding Intellectual Disability Transforms the Way We Read*. New York: New York University Press, 2016.

Bivens, Kristin Marie. "Rhetorical Ventriloquism, Earwitnessing, and Soundscapes in a Neonatal Intensive Care Unit (NICU)." *Rhetoric of Health and Medicine* 2, no 1. (2019): 1–32.

Blankmeyer Burke, Teresa. "Choosing Accommodations: Signed Language Interpreting and the Absence of Choice." *Kennedy Institute of Ethics Journal* 27, no. 2 (2017): 267–99.

Blankmeyer Burke, Teresa. "Teresa Blankmeyer Burke—Philosophy, Deaf Studies, Bioethics, Disability Studies," accessed January 31, 2020. https://teresablankmeyerburke.net/

Blankmeyer Burke, Teresa, and Brenda Nicodemus. "Coming out of the Hard of Hearing Closet: Reflections on a Shared Journey in Academia." *Disability Studies Quarterly* 33, no. 2 (2013).

Bogdan, Robert, with Martin Elks and James A. Knoll. *Picturing Disability: Beggar, Freak, Citizen, and other Photograph Rhetoric*. Syracuse, NY: Syracuse University Press, 2012.

Brekhus, Wayne H. *Culture and Cognition: Patterns in the Social Construction of Reality*. Cambridge, UK: Polity Press, 2015.

Brown, Kailyn. "Q&A: Porochista Khakpour's Long Struggle with Being *Sick*." *Los Angeles Times*, June 21, 2018. www.latimes.com

Brown, Nicole, and Jennifer Leigh, eds. *Ableism in Academia: Theorising Experiences of Disabilities and Chronic Illness in Higher Education*. London: UCL Press, 2020.

Brownlee, Mike. "City Reverses Stance on 'Deaf Child' Signage." *Daily Nonpareil*, February 28, 2010. https://nonpareilonline.com/

Brueggemann, Brenda Jo. "An Enabling Pedagogy: Meditations on Writing and Disability." *JAC: Journal of Composition Theory* 21, no. 4 (2001): 791–820.

Brueggemann, Brenda Jo. *Deaf Subjects: Between Identities and Places*. New York: New York University Press, 2009.

Brueggemann, Brenda Jo. *Lend Me Your Ear: Rhetorical Constructions of Deafness*. Washington, DC: Gallaudet University Press, 1999.

Brueggemann, Brenda Jo, and Stephanie L. Kerschbaum. "Disability: Representation, Disclosure, Access, and Interdependence." In *How to Build a Life in the Humanities*, edited by Greg Colón-Semenza and Garrett A. Sullivan Jr., 183–92. New York: Palgrave Macmillan, 2015.

Brune, Jeffrey A., and Daniel J. Wilson, eds. *Disability and Passing: Blurring the Lines of Identity*. Philadelphia: Temple University Press, 2013.

Burrows, Cedric. *Rhetorical Crossover: The Black Presence in White Culture*. Pittsburgh, PA: University of Pittsburgh Press, 2020.

Campt, Tina M. *Listening to Images*. Durham, NC: Duke University Press, 2017.

Canagarajah, Suresh. "Weaving the Text: Changing Literacy Practices and Orientations." *College English* 82, no. 1 (2019): 7–28.

Canguilhem, Georges. *The Normal and the Pathological*. Translated by Carolyn R. Fawcett. Boston: Massachusetts Institute of Technology Press, 1989.

Carter-Tod, Sheila, and Jennifer Sano-Franchini, eds. "Black Lives Matter and Anti-Racist Projects in Writing Program Administration." Special issue of *WPA: Writing Program Administration* 44, no. 3 (2021). http://wpacouncil.org/

Cedillo, Christina V. "What Does It Mean to Move? Race, Disability, and Critical Embodiment Pedagogy." *Composition Forum* 39 (2018). https://compositionforum.com/

Ceraso, Steph. "Sound Never Tasted So Good: 'Teaching' Sensory Rhetorics." *intermezzo* (2019). http://intermezzo.enculturation.net/

Ceraso, Steph. *Sounding Composition: Multimodal Pedagogies for Embodied Listening*. Pittsburgh, PA: University of Pittsburgh Press, 2018.

Chapple, Reshawna L., Binnae A. Bridwell, and Kishonna L. Gray. "Exploring Intersectional Identity in Black Deaf Women: The Complexity of the Lived Experience in College." *Affilia: Journal of Women and Social Work* 36, no. 4 (2021): 571–92.

Chen, Mel Y. *Animacies: Biopolitics, Racial Mattering, and Queer Affect*. Durham, NC: Duke University Press, 2012.

Clare, Eli. *Brilliant Imperfection: Grappling with Cure*. Durham, NC: Duke University Press, 2017.

Clare, Eli. *Exile and Pride: Disability, Queerness, and Liberation*. Cambridge, MA: South End Press, 1999.

Clark, Alex. "Porochista Khakpour, Author of *Sick*: 'It's More Convenient to Treat Patients as Crazy.'" *Guardian*, July 28, 2018. https://www.theguardian.com/

Connor, David J., Beth A. Ferri, and Subini A. Annamma, eds. *DisCrit: Disability Studies and Critical Race Theory in Education*. New York: Teachers College Press, 2016.

Cooper, Brittney. *Beyond Respectability: The Intellectual Thought of Race Women*. Urbana: University of Illinois Press, 2017.

Cooper, Marilyn M. *The Animal Who Writes: A Posthumanist Composition*. Pittsburgh, PA: University of Pittsburgh Press, 2019.

Couser, G. Thomas. *Recovering Bodies: Illness, Disability, and Life Writing*. Madison: University of Wisconsin Press, 1997.

Craig, Collin Lamont, and Staci Maree Perryman-Clark. "Troubling the Boundaries: (De)Constructing WPA Identities at the Intersection of Race and Gender." *WPA: Writing Program Administration* 34, no. 2 (2011): 37–58.

Craig, Sherri. "A Story-less Generation: Emergent WPAs of Color and the Loss of Identity through Absent Narratives." *WPA: Writing Program Administration* 39, no. 2 (2016): 16–20.

Crosby, Christina. *A Body, Undone: Living On after Great Pain*. New York: NYU Press, 2016.

Davila, Bethany. "Indexicality and 'Standard' Edited American English: Examining the Link between Conceptions of Standardness and Perceived Authorial Identity." *Written Communication* 29, no. 2 (2012): 180–207.

Davila, Bethany. "Standard English and Colorblindness in Composition Studies: Rhetorical Constructions of Racial and Linguistic Neutrality." *WPA: Writing Program Administration* 40, no. 2 (2017): 154–73.

Davis, Lennard J. *Enabling Acts: The Hidden Story of How the Americans with Disabilities Act Gave the Largest US Minority Its Rights*. Boston: Beacon Press, 2015.

Davis, Lennard J. *Enforcing Normalcy: Disability, Deafness, and the Body*. New York: Verso, 1995.

Day, Allyson. *The Political Economy of Stigma: HIV, Memoir, Medicine, and Crip Positionalities*. Columbus: Ohio State University Press, 2021.

Dingo, Rebecca. "Reevaluating Girls' Empowerment: Toward a Transnational Feminist Literacy." In *Circulation, Writing, and Rhetoric*, edited by Laurie E. Gries and Collin Gifford Brooke, 135–51. Logan: Utah State University Press, 2018.

Dolmage, Jay Timothy. *Academic Ableism: Disability and Higher Education*. Ann Arbor: University of Michigan Press, 2017.

Dolmage, Jay Timothy. *Disability Rhetoric*. Syracuse, NY: Syracuse University Press, 2014.

Dolmage, Jay Timothy. "Framing Disability, Developing Race: Photography as Eugenic Technology." *Enculturation*, March 11, 2014. https://www.enculturation.net/

Dolmage, Jay, and Stephanie L. Kerschbaum. "Wanted: Disabled Faculty Members." *Inside Higher Ed*, October 31, 2016. https://www.insidehighered.com/

Doubek, James. "Oklahoma City Police Fatally Shoot Deaf Man Despite Yells of 'He Can't Hear.'" National Public Radio, September 21, 2017. https://www.npr.org/

Dougher, Kelly. "How Not to Be a Dick to a Deaf Person." *xoJane*, May 29, 2013. https://web.archive.org/web/20170207010832/http://www.xojane.com/issues/how -not-to-be-a-dick-to-your-deaf-friend

Downey, Gregory J. *Closed Captioning: Subtitling, Stenography, and the Digital Convergence of Text with Television*. Baltimore, MD: Johns Hopkins University Press, 2008.

Dryer, Dylan B. "At a Mirror, Darkly: The Imagined Undergraduate Writers of Ten Novice Composition Instructors." *College Composition and Communication* 63, no. 3 (2012): 420–52.

Dunn, Dana S. *The Social Psychology of Disability*. Oxford: Oxford University Press, 2015.

Egner, Justine. "'The Disability Rights Community Was Never Mine': Neuroqueer Disidentification." *Gender and Society* 33, no. 1 (2019): 123–47.

Elman, Julie Passanante. "Policing at the Synapse: Ferguson, Race, and the Disability Politics of the Teen Brain." *Somatosphere: Science, Medicine, and Anthropology*, May 4, 2015. http://somatosphere.net/

Erevelles, Nirmala. *Disability and Difference in Global Contexts: Enabling a Transformative Body Politic*. New York: Palgrave Macmillan, 2011.

Ferguson, Roderick A. *The Reorder of Things: The University and Its Pedagogies of Minority Difference*. Minneapolis: University of Minnesota Press, 2012.

Fielder, Brigitte, and Jonathan Senchyne, eds. *Against a Sharp White Background: Infrastructures of African American Print*. Madison: University of Wisconsin Press, 2019.

Fink, Margaret. "Disabling Research Methods: Rights and Wrong Turns." Roundtable comments at the Society for Disability Studies, Atlanta, GA, June 10–13, 2015.

Flores, Lisa A. "Stoppage and the Racialized Rhetorics of Mobility." *Western Journal of Communication* 84, no. 3 (2020): 247–63.

Friedman, Asia. *Blind to Sameness: Sexpectations and the Social Construction of Male and Female Bodies*. Chicago: University of Chicago Press, 2013.

Friedman, Asia. "Cultural Blind Spots and Blind Fields: Collective Forms of Unawareness." In *The Oxford Handbook of Cognitive Sociology*, edited by Wayne H. Brekhus and Gabe Ignatow, 1–18. New York: Oxford University Press, 2019.

Friedner, Michele. "Biopower, Biosociality, and Community Formation: How Biopower Is Constitutive of the Deaf Community." *Sign Language Studies* 10, no. 3 (2010): 336–47.

Friedner, Michele, and Stefan Helmreich. "Sound Studies Meets Deaf Studies." *Senses & Society* 7, no. 1 (2012): 72–86.

Fritsch, Kelly. "The Neoliberal Circulation of Affects: Happiness, Accessibility, and the Capacitation of Disability as Wheelchair." *Health, Culture, and Society* 5, no. 1 (2013): 135–49.

Ganin, Netanel. "Disability in the Library of Congress Classification Scheme—Part 1." *I Never Metadata I Didn't Like*, August 16, 2015. https://inevermetadataididntlike.word press.com/2015/08/15/disability-in-the-library-of-congress-classification-scheme-part-1/

Ganin, Netanel. "Disability in the Library of Congress Classification Scheme—Part 2." *I Never Metadata I Didn't Like*, August 16, 2015. https://inevermetadataididntlike. wordpress.com/2015/08/16/disability-in-the-library-of-congress-classification-scheme -part-2/

Garland-Thomson, Rosemarie. *Extraordinary Bodies: Figuring Physical Disability in American Culture and Literature*. New York: Columbia University Press, 1997.

Garland-Thomson, Rosemarie. "Misfits: A Feminist Materialist Disability Concept." *Hypatia* 26, no. 3 (2011): 591–609.

Garland-Thomson, Rosemarie. *Staring: How We Look*. New York: Oxford University Press, 2009.

Garrison, Kevin. "Theorizing Lip Reading as Interface Design: The Gadfly in the Gaps." *Communication Design Quarterly Review* 6, no. 4 (2019): 24–34.

Gay, Roxane. *Hunger: A Memoir of My Body*. New York: Harper, 2017.

Genette, Gerard. *Paratexts: Thresholds of Interpretation*. New York: Cambridge University Press, 1997.

Georgakopoulou, Alexandra. *Small Stories, Interaction, and Identities*. Philadelphia: John Benjamins, 2007.

Glick, Megan H. *Infrahumanisms: Science, Culture, and the Making of Modern Non/ Personhood*. Durham, NC: Duke University Press, 2018.

Godfrey, Mollie, and Vershawn Ashanti Young, eds. *Neo-Passing: Performing Identity after Jim Crow*. Urbana: University of Illinois Press, 2018.

Goren, William D. *Understanding the Americans with Disabilities Act*. 3rd ed. Chicago: American Bar Association, 2010.

Grantham, Callum. "The Five Golden Rules of alt-text." *AbilityNet*, April 14, 2014. https://www.abilitynet.org.uk

Guffey, Elizabeth. *Designing Disability: Symbols, Space, and Society*. New York: Bloomsbury, 2018.

Gumbs, Alexis Pauline. "The Shape of My Impact." *Feminist Wire*, October 29, 2012. https://www.thefeministwire.com

Hames-García, Michael. *Identity Complex: Making the Case for Multiplicity*. Minneapolis: University of Minnesota Press, 2011.

Hammer, Gili. *Blindness through the Looking Glass: The Performance of Blindness, Gender, and the Sensory Body*. Ann Arbor: University of Michigan Press, 2019.

Hamraie, Aimi. *Building Access: Universal Design and the Politics of Disability*. Minneapolis: University of Minnesota Press, 2017.

Hamraie, Aimi, and Kelly Fritsch. "Crip Technoscience Manifesto." *Catalyst: Feminism, Theory, Technoscience* 5, no. 1 (2019): 1–34.

Harriet Tubman Collective. "Disability Solidarity: Completing the 'Vision for Black Lives.'" In *Disability Visibility: First Person Stories from the Twenty-first Century*, edited by Alice Wong, 236–42. New York: Vintage Books, 2020.

Hartman, Saidiya. "Venus in Two Acts." *Small Axe* 12, no. 2 (June 2008): 1–14.

Hauser, Peter C., Karen L. Finch, and Angela B. Hauser, eds. *Deaf Professionals and Designated Interpreters: A New Paradigm*. Washington, DC: Gallaudet University Press, 2008.

Hekman, Susan. *The Material of Knowledge: Feminist Disclosures*. Bloomington: Indiana University Press, 2010.

Helton, Laura E. "On Decimals, Catalogs, and Racial Imaginaries of Reading." *PMLA* 134, no. 1 (2019): 99–120.

Hendren, Sara. "An Icon Is a Verb: About the Project." The Accessible Icon Project, February 2016. www.accessibleicon.org.

Hitt, Allison. *Rhetorics of Overcoming: Rewriting Narratives of Disability and Accessibility in Writing Studies*. Urbana, IL: National Council of Teachers of English, 2021.

Hobbs, Allyson. *A Chosen Exile: A History of Racial Passing in American Life*. Cambridge, MA: Harvard University Press, 2014.

Hockenberry, John. *Moving Violations: War Zones, Wheel Chairs, and Declarations of Independence*. New York: Hyperion, 1995.

Hsu, V. Jo. "Reflection as Relationality: Rhetorical Alliances and Teaching Alternative Rhetorics." *College Composition and Communication* 70, no. 2 (2018): 142–68.

Hubrig, Adam, and Ruth Osorio, eds. "Enacting a Culture of Access in Our Conference Spaces." *College Composition and Communication* 72, no. 1 (2020): 87–117.

Inoue, Asao B. "Racism in Writing Programs and the CWPA." *Writing Program Administration* 40, no. 1 (2016): 134–54.

Inoue, Asao B., and Mya Poe, eds. *Race and Writing Assessment*. New York: Peter Lang, 2012.

Johnson, Harriet McBryde. *Too Late to Die Young: Nearly True Tales from a Life*. New York: Holt, 2005.

Johnson, Merri Lisa, and Robert McRuer. "Cripistemologies: Introduction," in "Cripistemologies: Part I," edited by Merri Lisa Johnson and Robert McRuer. Special issue of *Journal of Literary & Cultural Disability Studies* 8, no. 2 (2014): 127–47.

Kafer, Alison. *Feminist, Queer, Crip*. Bloomington: Indiana University Press, 2013.

Kahneman, Daniel. *Thinking, Fast and Slow*. New York: Farrar, Straus, and Giroux, 2011.

Kar Tang, Jasmine, Noro Andriamanalina, Sherri Craig, Collin Lamont Craig, Staci M. Perryman-Clark, Regina McManigell Grijalva, Genevieve García de Müeller, Cedric D. Burrows, James Chase Sanchez, and Tyler S. Branson. "Challenging Whiteness and/in Writing Program Administration and Writing Programs." *WPA: Writing Program Administration* 39, no. 2 (2016): 9–52.

Katz, Sarah. "Is There a Right Way to Be Deaf?" *New York Times*, November 7, 2019. https://www.nytimes.com

Kaul, Kate. "Risking Experience: Disability, Precarity, and Disclosure." In *Negotiating Disability: Disclosure and Higher Education*, edited by Stephanie L. Kerschbaum, Laura T. Eisenman, and James M. Jones, 171–87. Ann Arbor: University of Michigan Press, 2017.

Kennedy, Krista. "Being Seen Deaf; or, Pools as Borders." *Tendon: A Medical Humanities Creative Journal* 1 (2019). https://hopkinsmedicalhumanities.org/

Kennedy, Krista. "'I Forgot I'm Deaf!': Passing, Kairotic Space, and the Midcentury Cyborg Woman." *Rhetoric Society Quarterly* 50, no. 3 (2020): 184–93.

Kerschbaum, Stephanie L. "Anecdotal Relations: On Orienting to Disability in the Composition Classroom." *Composition Forum* 32 (Fall 2015). https://composition forum.com/

Kerschbaum, Stephanie L. "Disabled Faculty and Linguistic Agency." Modern Language Association Conference, Boston, MA, January 2013.

Kerschbaum, Stephanie L. "Exploring Discomfort Using Markers of Difference: Constructing Anti-Racist and Anti-Ableist Teaching Practices." In *Writing across Difference: Theory and Intervention*, edited by James Rushing Daniel, Katie Malcolm, and Candice Rai. 77–93. Logan: Utah State University Press, 2022.

Kerschbaum, Stephanie L. "On Rhetorical Agency and Disclosing Disability in Academic Writing." *Rhetoric Review* 33, no. 1 (2014): 55–71.

Kerschbaum, Stephanie L. "Sign Language Transcription and Qualitative Research Methodologies." In *Centering Diverse Bodyminds in Critical Qualitative Inquiry*, edited by Emily A. Nusbaum and Jessica Nina Lester, 49–61. New York: Routledge, 2021.

Kerschbaum, Stephanie L. "Signs of Disability, Disclosing." *enculturation* 30 (2019). www.enculturation.net

Kerschbaum, Stephanie L. *Toward a New Rhetoric of Difference*. Urbana, IL: National Council of Teachers of English, 2014.

Kerschbaum, Stephanie L., Laura T. Eisenman, and James M. Jones, eds. *Negotiating Disability: Disclosure and Higher Education*. Ann Arbor: University of Michigan Press, 2017.

Kerschbaum, Stephanie L., and Margaret Price. "Centering Disability in Qualitative Interviewing." *Research in the Teaching of English* 52, no. 1 (2017): 98–107.

Khakpour, Porochista. *Sick: A Memoir*. New York: Harper Perennial, 2018.

Khalifa, Ahmed. "Deaf Anxiety: What Is It and Why We Should Talk about It?" Hear Me Out!, September 27, 2019. https://hearmeoutcc.com

Kim, Eunjung. "Asexuality in Disability Narratives." *Sexualities* 14, no. 4 (2011): 479–93.

Kim, Eunjung. *Curative Violence: Rehabilitating Disability, Gender, and Sexuality in Modern Korea*. Durham, NC: Duke University Press, 2017.

Kim, Eunjung. "Unbecoming Human: An Ethics of Objects." *GLQ: A Journal of Lesbian and Gay Studies* 21, no. 2–3 (2015): 295–320.

Kim, Jina B. "Toward a Crip-of-Color Critique: Thinking with Minich's 'Enabling Whom?'" *Lateral: Journal of the Cultural Studies Association* 6, no. 1 (2017).

Kimmerer, Robin Wall. *Braiding Sweetgrass: Indigenous Wisdom, Scientific Knowledge, and the Teachings of Plants*. Minneapolis, MN: Milkweed Editions, 2013.

King, Lisa, Rose Gubele, and Joyce Rain Anderson, eds. *Survivance, Sovereignty, and Story: Teaching American Indian Rhetorics*. Logan: Utah State University Press, 2015.

Kleege, Georgina. "Aurality." In *Further Reading*, edited by Matthew Rubery and Leah Price, 206–12. New York: Oxford University Press, 2020.

Konrad, Annika. "Access Fatigue: The Rhetorical Work of Disability in Everyday Life." *College English* 83, no. 3 (2021): 179–99.

Konrad, Annika. "Reimagining Work: Normative Commonplaces and Their Effects on Accessibility in Workplaces." *Business and Professional Communications Quarterly* 81, no. 1 (2018): 123–41.

Kupetz, Joshua. "Disability Ecology and the Dematerialization of Literacy Disability Studies." In *The Matter of Disability: Materiality, Biopolitics, Crip Affect*, edited by David T. Mitchell, Susan Antebi, and Sharon L. Snyder, 48–66. Ann Arbor: University of Michigan Press, 2019.

Kuusisto, Stephen. "Intersection: New York City." In *Eavesdropping: A Life by Ear*. New York: Norton, 2006.

Kynard, Carmen. "Teaching while Black: Witnessing and Countering Disciplinary Whiteness, Racial Violence, and University Race-Management." *Literacy in Composition Studies* 3, no. 1 (2015): 1–20.

Labov, William, and Joshua Waletzky. "Narrative Analysis: Oral Versions of Personal Experience." *Journal of Narrative and Life History* 7, no. 1–4 (1997): 3–38.

Laymon, Kiese. *Heavy: An American Memoir*. New York: Scribners, 2018.

Lee, Robert, and Tristan Ahtone. "Land-Grab Universities." *High Country News* 52, no. 4 (March 30, 2020). https://www.hcn.org

Lewis, Talila "TL." "Stolen Bodies, Criminalized Minds, and Diagnosed Dissent: The Racist, Classist, Ableist Trappings of the Prison Industrial Complex." Longmore Lecture in Disability Studies, San Francisco State University, February 19, 2019. https://www.talilalewis.com

Lewis, Talila "TL," in community with Disabled Black and other negatively racialized people, especially Dustin Gibson. "January 2021 Working Definition of Ableism." Talila A. Lewis, accessed January 14, 2021. https://www.talilalewis.com/

Lindquist, Julie. *A Place to Stand: Politics and Persuasion in a Working-Class Bar*. New York: Oxford University Press, 2002.

Linett, Maren Tova. *Bodies of Modernism: Physical Disability in Transatlantic Modernist Literature*. Ann Arbor: University of Michigan Press, 2017.

Linton, Simi. *Claiming Disability: Knowledge and Identity*. New York: New York University Press, 1998.

Lukin, Josh. "Science Fiction, Affect, and Crip Self-Invention; or, How Philip K. Dick Made Me Disabled." In *Negotiating Disability: Disclosure and Higher Education*, edited by Stephanie L. Kerschbaum, Laura T. Eisenman, and James M. Jones, 227–42. Ann Arbor: University of Michigan Press, 2017.

Mairs, Nancy. *Waist-High in the World: A Life among the Nondisabled*. Boston: Beacon Press, 1996.

Manning, Erin, Brian Massumi, Jonas Fritsch, and Bodil Marie Stavning. "Affective Attunement in an Age of Catastrophe." *Peripeti*, June 6, 2012. https://www.peripeti.dk/

Martinez, Aja. *Counterstory: The Rhetoric and Writing of Critical Race Theory*. Urbana, IL: National Council of Teachers of English, 2020.

McHenry, Elizabeth. *Forgotten Readers: Recovering the Lost History of African American Literary Societies*. Durham, NC: Duke University Press, 2002.

McHenry, Elizabeth. "Toward a History of Access: The Case of Mary Church Terrell." *American Literary History* 19, no. 2 (2007): 381–401.

McKittrick, Katherine. *Dear Science and Other Stories*. Durham, NC: Duke University Press, 2021.

McKittrick, Katherine. "Yours in the Intellectual Struggle: Sylvia Wynter and the Realization of the Living." In *Sylvia Wynter: On Being Human as Praxis*, edited by Katherine McKittrick, 1–8. Durham, NC: Duke University Press, 2015.

Millett-Galant, Ann. *Re-Membering: Putting Mind and Body Back Together Following Traumatic Brain Injury*. Scotts Valley, CA: CreateSpace Independent Publishing Platform, 2013.

Mills, Charles W. "Materializing Race." In *Living Alterities: Phenomenology, Embodiment, and Race*, edited by Emily S. Lee, 19–41. Albany: State University of New York Press, 2014.

Mingus, Mia. "Reflections on an Opening: Disability Justice and Creating Collective Access in Detroit." Leaving Evidence, August 23, 2010, accessed February 10, 2021. https://leavingevidence.wordpress.com/

Minich, Julie Avril. "Enabling Whom? Critical Disability Studies Now." *Lateral: Journal of the Cultural Studies Association* 5, no. 1 (2016). https://csalateral.org/

Mishler, Elliot. *Research Interviewing: Context and Narrative*. Cambridge, MA: Harvard University Press, 1986.

Mitchell, David T., Susan Antebi, and Sharon L. Snyder. Introduction to *The Matter of Disability: Materiality, Biopolitics, Crip Affect*, edited by David T. Mitchell, Susan Antebi, and Sharon L. Snyder, 1–36. Ann Arbor: University of Michigan Press, 2019.

Mitchell, David T., and Sharon L. Snyder. "Posthumanist T4 Memory." In *The Matter of Disability: Materiality, Biopolitics, Crip Affect*, edited by David T. Mitchell, Susan Antebi, and Sharon L. Snyder, 249–72. Ann Arbor: University of Michigan Press, 2019.

Moody-Turner, Shirley. "'Dear Doctor Du Bois': Anna Julia Cooper, W. E. B. Du Bois, and the Gender Politics of Black Publishing." *MELUS* 40, no. 3 (2015): 47–68.

Moody-Turner, Shirley. "Prospects for the Study of Anna Julia Cooper." *Resources for American Literary Study* 40 (2018): 1–29.

Moore, Leroy F., Jr., Talila A. "TL" Lewis, Lydia X. Z. Brown, and the Harriet Tubman Collective. "Accountable Reporting on Disability, Race, and Police Violence: A Community Response to the 'Ruderman White Paper on Media Coverage on Use of Force and Disability.'" Tumblr, June 1, 2018. https://harriettubmancollective.tumblr.com/

Morrison, Aimée. "(Un)Reasonable, (Un)Necessary, and (In)Appropriate: Biographic Mediation of Neurodivergence in Academic Accommodations." *Biography* 42, no. 3 (2019): 693–719.

Mullaney, Clare. "Dickinson, Disability, and a Crip Editorial Practice." In *The New Dickinson Studies*, edited by Michelle Kohler, 280–98. New York: Cambridge University Press, 2019.

Mullaney, Clare. "'Not to Discover Weakness Is the Artifice of Strength': Emily Dickinson, Constraint, and a Disability Poetics." *J19: The Journal of 19th Century Americanists* 7, no. 1 (2019): 49–81.

Muñoz, José Esteban. *Disidentifications: Queers of Color and the Performance of Politics.* Minneapolis: University of Minnesota Press, 1999.

Murphy, Michelle. *Sick Building Syndrome and the Problem of Uncertainty: Environmental Politics, Technoscience, and Women Workers.* Durham, NC: Duke University Press, 2006.

Nam, Susie E. "Making Visible the Dead Bodies in the Room: Women of Color/QPOC in Academia." In *Presumed Incompetent II: Race, Class, Power, and Resistance of Women in Academia,* edited by Yolanda Flores Niemann, Gabriella Gutiérrez y Muhs, and Carmen G. González, 171–79. Logan: Utah State University Press, 2020.

Nishida, Akemi. "Neoliberal Academia and a Critique from Disability Studies." In *Occupying Disability: Critical Approaches to Community, Justice, and Decolonizing Disability,* edited by Pamela Block, Devva Kasnitz, Akemi Nishida, and Nick Pollard, 145–57. New York: Springer, 2016.

Noble, Safiya Umoja. *Algorithms of Oppression: How Search Engines Reinforce Racism.* New York: New York University Press, 2018.

Nusbaum, Emily, and Jessica Nina Lester, eds. *Centering Diverse Bodyminds in Critical Qualitative Inquiry.* New York: Routledge, 2021.

Nye, Coleman. "Porochista Khakpour's *Sick*." In *Disability Experiences: Memoirs, Autobiographies, and Other Personal Narratives,* edited by G. Thomas Couser and Susannah B. Mintz, vol. 2: 684–88. Farmington Hills, MI: Macmillan Reference, 2019.

Ochs, Elinor, and Lisa Capps. *Living Narrative: Creating Lives in Everyday Storytelling.* Cambridge, MA: Harvard University Press, 2001.

Okun, Tema, et al. "(Divorcing) White Supremacy Culture: Coming Home to Who We Really Are." DRWorksBook, accessed July 15, 2021. https://www.whitesuprem acyculture.info

Ore, Ersula J. *Lynching: Violence, Rhetoric, and American Identity.* Jackson: University Press of Mississippi, 2019.

Oxford English Dictionary, s.v. "dis-, prefix," accessed January 22, 2020. https://www .oed.com

Park, Joseph Sung-Yun, and Mary Bucholtz. "Public Transcripts: Entextualization and Linguistic Representation in Institutional Contexts." *Text and Talk* 29, no. 5 (2009): 485–502.

Perryman-Clark, Staci M., and Collin Lamont Craig, eds., *Black Perspectives in Writing Program Administration: From the Margins to the Center.* Urbana, IL: National Council of Teachers of English, 2019.

Pickens, Therí Alyce. *Black Madness :: Mad Blackness.* Durham, NC: Duke University Press, 2019.

Pickens, Therí Alyce. *New Body Politics: Narrating Arab and Black Identity in the Contemporary United States.* New York: Routledge, 2014.

Piepzna-Samarasinha, Leah Lakshmi. *Care Work: Dreaming Disability Justice*. Vancouver, BC, Canada: Arsenal Pulp Press, 2018.

Piepzna-Samarasinha, Leah Lakshmi. "How Disabled Mutual Aid Is Different Than Abled Mutual Aid." Disability Visibility Project, October 2021, accessed November 10, 2021. https://disabilityvisibilityproject.com/

Powell, Malea. "Listening to Ghosts: An Alternative (Non)Argument." In *Alt Dis: Alternative Discourses in the Academy*, edited by Christopher Schroeder, Helen Fox, and Patricia Bizzell, 11–22. Portsmouth, NH: Boynton/Cook, 2002.

Powell, Malea, Daisy Levy, Andrea Riley-Mukavetz, Marilee Brooks-Gillies, Maria Novotny, Jennifer Fisch-Ferguson, and the Cultural Rhetorics Theory Lab. "Our Story Begins Here: Constellating Cultural Rhetorics." *enculturation*, no. 18 (2014). https://www.enculturation.net

Prahlad, Anand. *The Secret Life of a Black Aspie: A Memoir*. Fairbanks: University of Alaska Press, 2017.

Price, Margaret. "The Bodymind Problem and the Possibilities of Pain." *Hypatia* 30, no. 1 (2015): 268–84.

Price, Margaret. "Disability Studies Methodology: Explaining Ourselves to Ourselves." In *Practicing Research in Writing Studies: Reflexive and Ethically Responsive Research*, edited by Katrina M. Powell and Pamela Takayoshi, 159–86. New York: Hampton Press, 2012.

Price, Margaret. *Mad at School: Rhetorics of Mental Disability and Academic Life*. Ann Arbor: University of Michigan Press, 2011.

Price, Margaret. "Time Harms: Disabled Faculty Navigating the Accommodations Loop." *South Atlantic Quarterly* 120, no. 2 (2021): 257–77.

Price, Margaret. "Un/Shared Space: The Dilemma of Inclusive Architecture." *Disability, Space, Architecture*, edited by Jos Boys, 149–67. New York: Routledge, 2017.

Price, Margaret, and Stephanie L. Kerschbaum. "Stories of Methodology: Interviewing Sideways, Crooked, and Crip." *Canadian Journal of Disability Studies* 5, no. 3 (2016): 18–56.

Price, Margaret, Mark S. Salzer, Amber O'Shea, and Stephanie L. Kerschbaum, "Disclosure of Mental Disability by College and University Faculty: The Negotiation of Accommodations, Supports, and Barriers." *Disability Studies Quarterly* 37, no. 2 (2017). http://dsq-sds.org/

Puar, Jasbir K. *The Right to Maim: Debility, Capacity, Disability*. Durham, NC: Duke University Press, 2017.

Rak, Julie. *Boom! Manufacturing Memoir for the Popular Market*. Waterloo, ON, Canada: Wilfred Laurier University Press, 2013.

Reeb, Celeste. "[This Closed Captioning Is Brought to You by Compulsive Heterosexuality/Able-bodiedness]." *Disability Studies Quarterly* 39, no. 3 (2019). https://dsq-sds.org/

Restaino, Jessica. *Surrender: Feminist Rhetoric and Ethics in Love and Illness*. Carbondale: Southern Illinois University Press, 2019.

Richardson, Elaine. *From PHD to PhD: How Education Saved My Life.* Philadelphia: New City Community Press, 2013.

Riley-Mukavetz, Andrea. "Developing a Relational Scholarly Practice: Snakes, Dreams, and Grandmothers." *College Composition and Communication* 71, no. 4 (2020): 545–65.

Robillard, Amy E. "Seeking Adequate Rhetorical Witnesses for Life Writing." *Rhetoric Society Quarterly* 49, no. 2 (2019): 185–92.

Rodas, Julia Miele. *Autistic Disturbances: Theorizing Autism Poetics from the* DSM *to Robinson Crusoe.* Foreword by Remi Yergeau. Ann Arbor: University of Michigan Press, 2018.

Sacks, Harvey, Emmanuel A. Schegloff, and Gail Jefferson. "A Simplest Systematics for the Organization of Turn-Taking for Conversation." *Language* 50, no. 4 (1974): 696–735.

Samuels, Ellen. *Fantasies of Identification: Disability, Gender, Race.* New York: New York University Press, 2014.

Samuels, Ellen. "My Body, My Closet." *GLQ: A Journal of Lesbian and Gay Studies* 9, no. 1–2 (2003): 233–55.

Samuels, Ellen. "Passing, Coming Out, and Other Magical Acts." In *Negotiating Disability: Disclosure and Higher Education,* edited by Stephanie L. Kerschbaum, Laura T. Eisenman, and James M. Jones, 15–24. Ann Arbor: University of Michigan Press, 2017.

Sánchez, María Carla, and Linda Schlossberg, eds. *Passing: Identity and Interpretation in Sexuality, Race, and Religion.* New York: New York University Press, 2001.

Sanchez, Rebecca. *Deafening Modernism: Embodied Language and Visual Poetics in American Literature.* New York: New York University Press, 2015.

Sanchez, Rebecca. "Doing Disability with Others." In *Negotiating Disability: Disclosure and Higher Education,* edited by Stephanie L. Kerschbaum, Laura T. Eisenman, and James M. Jones, 211–26. Ann Arbor: University of Michigan Press, 2017.

Sanchez, Rebecca. "'Human Bodies Are Words': Towards a Theory of Non-Verbal Voice." *CEA Critic* 73, no. 3 (2011): 33–47.

Sanchez, Rebecca. "Linguistic Othering." Keynote presentation, The Paradox of the Other conference, Brooklyn College, Brooklyn, NY, May 5, 2018.

Savageau, Cheryl. *Out of the Crazywoods.* Lincoln: University of Nebraska Press, 2020.

Savitz, Harriet May. *Wheelchair Champions: A History of Wheelchair Sports.* New York: Crowell, 1978.

Schalk, Sami. *Bodyminds Reimagined: (Dis)ability, Race, and Gender in Black Women's Speculative Fiction.* Durham, NC: Duke University Press, 2018.

Schalk, Sami. "Coming to Claim Crip: Disidentifying with Disability Studies." *Disability Studies Quarterly* 33, no. 2 (2013). https://dsq-sds.org/

Schalk, Sami, and Jina B. Kim. "Integrating Race, Transforming Feminist Disability Studies." *Signs: A Journal of Women in Culture and Society* 46, no. 1 (2020): 31–55.

Schiffrin, Deborah. *Discourse Markers.* New York: Cambridge University Press, 1987.

Schnitzer, Anna Ercoli, and Bonnie A. Dede. *Diversity Includes Disability: Perspectives on the U-M Council for Disability Concerns*. Ann Arbor: Michigan Publishing, University of Michigan Library, 2018. http://dx.doi.org/10.3998/mpub.9997270

Seidman, Irving. *Interviewing as Qualitative Research: A Guide for Researchers in Education and the Social Sciences*. 3rd edition. New York: Teachers College Press, 2006.

Shomura, Chad. "Exploring the Promise of New Materialisms." *Lateral: Journal of the Cultural Studies Association* 6, no. 1 (2017). https://csalateral.org/

Siebers, Tobin. *Disability Theory*. Ann Arbor: University of Michigan Press, 2008.

Siebers, Tobin. "Returning the Social to the Social Model." In *The Matter of Disability: Materiality, Biopolitics, Crip Affect*, edited by David T. Mitchell, Susan Antebi, and Sharon L. Snyder, 39–47. Ann Arbor: University of Michigan Press, 2019.

Sign Language ASL Dictionary, accessed January 25, 2021. https://www.handspeak.com

Silverman, Gillian. "Neurodiversity and the Revision of Book History." *PMLA* 131, no. 2 (2016): 307–23.

Sins Invalid. *Skin, Tooth, and Bone: The Basis of Movement Is Our People; A Disability Justice Primer*. 2nd ed. 2018. https://www.sinsinvalid.org/

Smith, David Harry, and Jean F. Andrews. "Deaf and Hard of Hearing Faculty in Higher Education: Enhancing Access, Equity, Policy, and Practice." *Disability and Society* 30, no. 10 (2015): 1521–36.

Snorton, C. Riley. *Black on Both Sides: A Racial History of Trans Identity*. Minneapolis: University of Minnesota Press, 2017.

Stremlau, Tonya. "Deaf Pedestrians." 241 Mom, April 9, 2013, accessed August 9, 2018. www.241mom.wordpress.com/

Sue, Derald Wing, Christina M. Capodilupo, Gina C. Torino, Jennifer M. Bucceri, Aisha M. B. Holder, Kevin L. Nadal, and Marta Esquilin. "Racial Microaggressions in Everyday Life: Implications for Clinical Practice." *American Psychologist* 62, no. 4 (2007): 271–86.

Taylor, Sunaura. *Beasts of Burden: Animal and Disability Liberation*. New York: New Press, 2017.

Titchkosky, Tanya. *The Question of Access: Disability, Space, Meaning*. Toronto: University of Toronto Press, 2011.

Towner, Emil B. "Danger in Public Spaces: Strengths and Limitations of Image- and Text-Based Warning Signs." *Business and Professional Communication Quarterly* 82, no. 1 (2019): 53–73.

Tullivan, Tipsy. "Tips for Writers by Tipsy Tullivan." YouTube, accessed January 11, 2022. https://www.youtube.com/channel/UCwfcYz-fiPjqoU6v-fevOMQ

University of Illinois at Urbana-Champaign. "Athletics: Disability Resources." Division of Disability Resources and Educational Services, accessed January 28, 2020. https://www.disability.illinois.edu/

University of Michigan. "Americans with Disabilities Act (ADA)." College of Literature, Science, and the Arts, accessed January 24, 2021. https://lsa.umich.edu/

Urban, Greg. "Entextualization, Replication, and Power." In *Natural Histories of Discourse*, edited by Michael Silverstein and Greg Urban, 21–44. Chicago: University of Chicago Press, 1996.

Valentine, David. *Imagining Transgender: An Ethnography of a Category*. Durham, NC: Duke University Press, 2007.

Vance, Mary Lee, ed. *Disabled Faculty and Staff in a Disabling Society: Multiple Identities in Higher Education*. Huntersville, NC: AHEAD, 2007.

Vest, Jennifer Lisa. "What Doesn't Kill You: Existential Luck, Postracial Racism, and the Subtle and Not So Subtle Ways the Academy Keeps Women of Color Out." *Seattle Journal for Social Justice* 12, no. 2 (2013): 471–518.

Vidali, Amy. "The Biggest Little Ways toward Access: Thinking with Disability in Site-Specific Rhetorical Work." *Review of Communication* 20, no. 2 (2020): 161–69.

Vidali, Amy. "Disabling Writing Program Administration." *Journal of the Council of Writing Program Administrators* 38, no. 2 (2015): 32–55.

Vidali, Amy. "Hysterical Again: The Gastrointestinal Woman in Medical Discourse." *Journal of Medical Humanities* 34, no. 1 (March 2013): 33–57.

Vidali, Amy. "Out of Control: Rhetorics of Gastrointestinal Disorder." *Disability Studies Quarterly* 30, no. 3/4 (Summer/Fall 2010). https://dsq-sds.org/

Vidali, Amy. "Seeing What We Know: Disability and Theories of Metaphor." *Journal of Literary & Cultural Disability Studies* 4, no. 1 (2010): 33–54.

Vidali, Amy, and Griffin Keedy. "Productive Chaos: Disability, Advising, and the Writing Process." *Praxis: A Writing Center Journal* 14, no. 1 (2016): 21–26.

Vieira, Kate. "What Happens When Texts Fly." *College English* 82, no. 1 (2019): 77–95.

Villanueva, Victor. *Bootstraps: From an American Academic of Color*. Urbana, IL: National Council of Teachers of English, 1993.

Villanueva, Victor. "Memoria Is a Friend of Ours: On the Discourse of Color." *College English* 67, no. 1 (2004): 9–19.

Virdi, Jaipreet. *Hearing Happiness: Deafness Cures in History*. Chicago: University of Chicago Press, 2020.

Virdi, Jaipreet. "Materializing User Identities through Disability Technologies." In *Making Disability Modern: Design Histories*, edited by Bess Williamson and Elizabeth Guffey, 225–41. New York: Bloomsbury, 2020.

Waite, Stacey. *Teaching Queer: Radical Possibilities for Writing and Knowing*. Pittsburgh, PA: University of Pittsburgh Press, 2017.

Wald, Gayle. *Crossing the Line: Racial Passing in Twentieth-Century U.S. Literature and Culture*. Durham, NC: Duke University Press, 2000.

WebAIM: Web Accessibility in Mind, accessed January 29, 2020. https://webaim.org/

Williamson, Bess. *Accessible America: A History of Disability and Design*. New York: New York University Press, 2019.

WisDOT Research & Library Unit. "Effectiveness of 'Children at Play' Warning Signs." Wisconsin Department of Transportation, September 25, 2007. 54.172.27.91/transportation/signs/ChildrenWarningSigns_TSR_2007.pdf

Wong, Alice. Disability Visibility Project, accessed December 30, 2020. https://disabilityvisibilityproject.com/

Wong, Alice, ed. *Disability Visibility: First-Person Stories from the Twenty-first Century.* New York: Vintage, 2020.

Woodcock, Kathryn, Meg J. Rohan, and Linda Campbell. "Equitable Representation of Deaf People in Mainstream Academia: Why Not?" *Higher Education* 53 (2007): 359–79.

Wortham, Stanton. "Interactional Positioning and Narrative Self-Construction." *Narrative Inquiry* 10, no. 1 (2000): 157–84.

Wortham, Stanton. *Narratives in Action: A Strategy for Research and Analysis.* New York: Teachers College Press, 2001.

Yergeau, Remi. *Authoring Autism: On Rhetoric and Neurological Queerness.* Durham, NC: Duke University Press, 2017.

Yergeau, Remi. "Creating a Culture of Access in Writing Program Administration." *WPA: Writing Program Administration* 40, no. 1 (2016): 155–65.

Yergeau, Remi. "Disable All the Things." Keynote Address, Computers and Writing Conference, Washington State University, Pullman, Washington, June 6, 2014.

Yergeau, Remi. "Rehabilitation ≠ what we do," in Remi Yergeau et al., "Multimodality in Motion." *Kairos: A Journal of Rhetoric, Technology, and Pedagogy* 18, no. 1 (2013). http://kairos.technorhetoric.net/

Yergeau, Remi, Elizabeth Brewer, Stephanie Kerschbaum, Sushil Oswal, Margaret Price, Cynthia Selfe, and Franny Howes. "Multimodality in Motion." *Kairos: A Journal of Rhetoric, Technology, and Pedagogy* 18, no. 1 (2013). http://kairos.tech norhetoric.net/

Yoshino, Kenji. *Covering: The Hidden Assault on Our Civil Rights.* New York: Random House, 2006.

Zdenek, Sean. *Reading Sounds: Closed-Caption Media and Popular Culture.* Chicago: University of Chicago Press, 2015.

Zerubavel, Eviatar. *Hidden in Plain Sight: The Social Structure of Irrelevance.* New York: Oxford University Press, 2015.

Zerubavel, Eviatar. *Taken for Granted: The Remarkable Power of the Unremarkable.* Princeton, NJ: Princeton University Press, 2018.

INDEX

Page numbers in italics indicate Figures

ABOUT THE AUTHOR

STEPHANIE L. KERSCHBAUM is Associate Professor of English at the University of Washington. She is the author of *Toward a New Rhetoric of Difference*, which won the 2015 Advancement of Knowledge Award from the Conference on College Composition and Communication, and coeditor of *Negotiating Disability: Disclosure and Higher Education*.

www.ingramcontent.com/pod-product-compliance
Lightning Source LLC
Chambersburg PA
CBHW020251030426
42336CB00010B/708